Mood Disorders

T0136272

Mood Disorders: Practical Issues in Diagnosis and Management provides cutting edge knowledge about the diagnosis and treatment of major mood disorders, namely major depressive disorder and bipolar disorder. Covering diagnosis, differentiating features, and illness course and trajectories of principal mood disorders, Dr. Ather Muneer provides essential information in a succinct and practical manner, while highlighting significant new findings in the area. This book will help a broad range of mental health professionals better treat the millions of people with mood disorders across the globe.

Dr. Ather Muneer, MD, is assistant professor of psychiatry at the Islamic International Medical College, Riphah International University, Islamabad. He has published papers in numerous journals, and is a member of the Pakistan Psychiatric Society and the European Psychiatric Association.

Mood Disorders
Practical Issues in Diagnosis and Management

By Dr. Ather Muneer

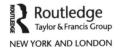

Routledge
Taylor & Francis Group

NEW YORK AND LONDON

First published 2018
by Routledge
711 Third Avenue, New York, NY 10017

and by Routledge
2 Park Square, Milton Park, Abingdon, Oxon, OX14 4RN

Routledge is an imprint of the Taylor & Francis Group, an informa business

Library of Congress Cataloging-in-Publication Data
A catalog record for this book has been requested

ISBN: 978-1-138-55449-8 (hbk)
ISBN: 978-1-138-55450-4 (pbk)
ISBN: 978-1-315-14934-9 (ebk)

Typeset in Goudy
by Out of House Publishing

Contents

List of Figures

List of Tables

1 Major Depressive Disorder and Bipolar Disorder

Introduction

According to the Diagnostic and Statistical Manual of Mental Disorders – 5th Edition (DSM-5) major mood disorders are classified into major depressive disorder (MDD) and bipolar disorder (BD). More than a century ago, the German psychiatrist Emil Kraepelin categorized major mental disorders into "manic depressive insanity" and "dementia praecox". The former was reconceptualized as a recurrent illness exemplified by repeated depressive and manic episodes while the latter was replaced by "schizophrenia", a word coined by the Swiss psychologist Eugene Bleuler and typified as a non-affective psychosis epitomized by delusions, hallucinations, blunting of affect and loss of motivation.[1] In the current rendition of DSM-5, MDD and BD are described under separate rubrics as these mood disorders are presently considered to have distinct etiology, pathogenesis, course and therapeutic connotations.

Major mood disorders are highly prevalent conditions affecting up to 20% of the general population.[2] Individuals of both sexes are afflicted, onset is usually in teenage years or early adulthood and the disorders follow a relapsing and remitting course throughout life. All the current treatments are palliative rather than curative in nature, and while the modern psychopharmacological agents have improved safety and efficacy, these still impose a huge burden with respect to adverse effects. Consequently, compliance is low and relapse rate is high with resultant impairment in the biopsychosocial realms of functioning.[3] Affective disorders are a leading cause of morbidity and mortality, since these are regarded as systemic ailments and are very often associated with such comorbid conditions as diabetes mellitus, cardiovascular diseases, auto immune disorders and endocrine disturbances.[4] The majority of people who commit suicide have an underlying mood disorder, and new data suggest that the incidence of this condition is on the rise across the world.[5] Because of these reasons World Health Organization statistics show that mood disorders are an important source of disability and death globally.[6] Therefore, in the light of such considerations it is crucial that physicians in general and mental health professionals in particular, have an adequate understanding of these very common psychiatric conditions.

Signs and Symptoms

Historical development in the nosology of mood disorders has led to their categorization into unipolar depression and BD. Essentially these are distinct conditions with different genetic underpinnings and disparate illness trajectory, progression and outcome. In essence, MDD is typified by recurrent depressive exacerbations without a lifetime history of hypomanic or manic episodes, whereas BD patients fluctuate between the opposite mood states of depression and mania.[7]

Major Depressive Episode

A major depressive episode (MDE) is signified by the presence of low mood and loss of pleasure in day-to-day activities, aptly termed anhedonia. The latter represents a distinct emotional tone in the patients, wherein they lose interest in the usual activities and no longer experience pleasure in things they previously found enjoyable. The cognitive process in MDE is exemplified by excessive guilt and self-blame, thoughts of helplessness and hopelessness and suicidal ideation. Disruption in the circadian rhythm is evident as sleep disturbance, with early morning wakening characterizing the more severe, melancholic form of MDD. There is usually decreased appetite and weight loss, but patients with "atypical depression" can have reverse vegetative disturbance with hypersomnia, increased food intake and weight gain. Subjects who have MDEs experience excessive mental and physical fatigue, loss of energy and tiredness and also complain of difficulty in concentration and indecisiveness. Further, they may show psychomotor retardation or agitation. Recurrent suicidal ideation and psychomotor agitation accompanying a low mood predisposes MDD patients to self-harm and attempted or completed suicide.[8] While the duration criteria stipulate a minimum period of two weeks, in the usual scenario patients are symptomatic for months before they seek medical help. As can be construed from the abovementioned facts, an MDE is a serious ailment which can prove fatal if there is delay in diagnosis and treatment. The vast majority of patients with MDD follow a relapsing and remitting course, and while it is possible to have a single lifetime MDE, this is the exception rather than the rule.[9]

Manic Episode

A manic episode is the *sine qua non* of BD and patients typically present with elevated or expansive mood. They have raised self-esteem and express grandiose ideas, which in the case of psychotic mania can be of delusional intensity. Subjectively, patients experience racing thoughts and objectively this is manifested as pressure of speech and flight of ideas. They have boosted energy levels and show increase in goal-directed activities; coupled with this is a decreased need for sleep. In severe mania, the patient is on the go most of the time, has boundless energy and feels rested after only a few hours of sleep. These subjects exhibit overindulgence in pleasurable activities and become part of risky ventures with high potential for harmful social consequences. Some examples are buying sprees, sexual indiscretions, and alcohol and substance abuse. A manic patient requires urgent treatment and is often in need of psychiatric hospitalization. Whereas the duration criteria stipulate a period of disturbance spanning one week, if hospitalization is mandated then a manic episode can be diagnosed with any period of mood disturbance.[10] The core symptoms of a hypomanic episode are essentially analogous to a manic episode, with the caveat that severe psychosocial disruption is not evident and emergency hospitalization is not needed.[11] Only four days of mood disturbance is sufficient to diagnose a hypomanic episode and, while the disorder is subtle in presentation, it is often part of chronic affective instability in bipolar spectrum disorders.

Mixed States

Mood symptoms can manifest in numerous ways and typical presentations are seen in only a minority of patients. A common clinical occurrence is the presence of mixed affective states, which can afflict people with both MDD and BD. The current conceptualization of mixed states posits that symptoms of opposite mood polarity are attendant in patients with major mood disorders. It is estimated that up to 40% of bipolar patients may be afflicted in this manner, while concurrent presence of hypomanic or manic symptoms in MDD is being increasingly recognized.[12] In essence, this implies that patients with manic or hypomanic episodes have coexisting depressive symptoms and vice versa. The clinical significance of mixed states is manifold. Firstly, the clinician should be cognizant of their occurrence and be on the lookout for the presence of mixed affective manifestations in patients with mood disorders. Secondly, it should be realized that repeated episodes of similar polarity occur, such that patients with mixed episodes tend to have the same exacerbations in the course of their illness. Thirdly, mixed episodes signify a more severe illness trajectory marked by treatment resistance, greater neuropsychiatric comorbidities and higher risk of suicide. Lastly, polypharmacy is the rule rather than the exception in the management of these cases and there is consequential patient noncompliance from medication adverse effects.[13]

Figure 1.1 is an illustrative rendition of the different mood states as envisaged in DSM-5. Table 1.1 recapitulates the main affective states as encountered in discrete mood episodes.

Diagnosis of Mood Disorders

Major mood disorders are represented by MDD and BD, and modern understanding informs us that these are systemic diseases with heterogeneous presentations. In the wake of this perception it is imperative that the treating

Manic/hypomanic episode	Depressive episode	Episode with mixed features
• elevated/expansive mood • inflated self-esteem/grandiosity • overtalkativeness/pressure of speech • flight of ideas/increased rate of thinking • enhanced energy/purposeful activities • increased involvement in activities with high risk of harmful consequences • less need for sleep	• prominent low mood • lack of pleasure in activities which were previously enjoyable • ↑ or ↓ weight • ↑ or ↓ sleep • psychic/motor agitation/retardation • ↓ energy • thoughts of worthlessness or guilt • ↓ concentration/indecisiveness • ideas of self-harm/suicidal attempt	• three or more manic/hypomanic symptoms in an MDE - BD type I - BD type II - MDD • three or more depressive symptoms in a manic or hypomanic episode - BD type I - BD type II

Figure 1.1 Diagnostic criteria for manic, depressive and mixed states according to DSM-5

As opposed to previous editions, in DSM-5 the specifier "with mixed features" is used for manic, hypomanic or depressive episodes in bipolar spectrum and major depressive disorders. The term "mixed episode" employed in the setting of BD type I has been discontinued in DSM-5.

BD – bipolar disorder; MDD – major depressive disorder; MDE – major depressive episode

physician realizes that he or she is, in fact, seeing a general ailment which has physical as well as psychological sequelae. From this perspective patients with chronic mood disorders must be considered to be prone to such complications as the metabolic syndrome, diabetes mellitus, and cardiovascular and other morbidities, and appropriate screening with physical examinations and directed laboratory investigations should be instituted at every follow-up visit.[14]

In addition, the following concerns are pertinent:

1) The onset is usually in adolescence or early adulthood.
2) Nonetheless, the symptomatic young person can present in a variety of ways such as conduct disorder, attention deficit hyperactivity disorder, anxiety spectrum disorders and substance use disorders.
3) As a result, the actual diathesis masquerades and the real diagnosis may be delayed.
4) Application of inappropriate and inadequate treatment measures leads to numerous complications in the psychological and social spheres of functioning.

Table 1.1 Diagnostic features of different affective states according to DSM-5

Symptom domain	Hypo/manic episode	Depressive episode	Episode with mixed features
Subjective mood	Elated	Depressed	Varies
Hedonic tone	↑involvement in pleasurable activities	Anhedonia	Mixture of both
Thought content	Grandiose	Worthlessness/ guilt	Varies
Talk	↑in rate, rhythm and volume	↓in rate, rhythm and volume	Incongruent e.g. depressed mood with pressure of speech
Behavior	Risky behaviors	Suicidal acts	Contrasting e.g. elevated mood with suicidal ideation
Energy	↑	↓	↑↓
Sleep	↓need for sleep	Early morning wakening	Severely disturbed
Thoughts	Racing thoughts	Difficulty in thinking/ concentration	Incongruent e.g. depressed mood with racing thoughts
Appetite/weight	Disrupted meal schedule	↓	Severe disruption
Duration	Hypomania – 4 days; mania – 7 days	14 days	Duration criteria no longer apply
Minimum criteria for mixed episode	Three depressive features in hypomanic or manic episode	Three manic features in a depressive episode	Mixed hypomania – BD type I or II Mixed mania – BD type I MDE with mixed features – BD type I or II/ MDD
Functioning	Hypomania – impaired but does not require hospitalization Mania – severely impaired/ may need hospitalization	Impaired according to degree – mild/ moderate/severe	Varies according to diagnosis

BD – bipolar disorder; MDD – major depressive disorder; MDE – major depressive episode

5) Persistent symptomatic state is detrimental to the young patient's physical and psychological well-being with multiple adverse consequences such as academic or occupational failure, substance dependence and breakdown in social relationships.
6) Repeated failures are very damaging to the patient's self-esteem and the ensuing vicious cycle causes an ever decreasing level of functioning in daily affairs.

With these caveats in mind, it is necessary that mental health professionals take an inclusive approach and provide the needed care at each level so patients with major mood disturbances can maintain autonomy and control over their affairs.[15] Figure 1.2 gives a schematic depiction of the pernicious nature of mood disorders and clarifies that a comprehensive approach is required for the proper treatment of these conditions.

Major Depressive Disorder

This disorder can be conceptualized as unipolar depression and is typified by recurrent MDEs. A lifetime episode of hypomania would change the diagnosis to BD type II, while the occurrence of a single manic episode would convert it to BD type I. In MDD, the MDE must arise de novo and not be secondary to substance abuse or a physical illness. While the onset can be at any time

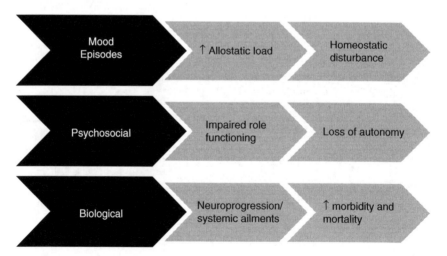

Figure 1.2 The pernicious nature of mood disorders

Mood disorders, whether MDD or BD, are conceptualized as very serious conditions with profound consequences in the biopsychosocial spheres of functioning. Repeated affective episodes increase "wear and tear" in the body with increased allostatic load. The resulting homeostatic imbalance has a pervasive negative effect with such consequences as cognitive impairment, physical comorbidities, and role impairment with eventual loss of self-independence.

from childhood to old age, the disorder usually first occurs in young adulthood. Whereas it is possible to have a single lifetime episode of major depression, the majority of cases follow a recurrent pattern. The course can be characterized as relapsing and remitting, and during periods of remission the patients may be entirely symptom free or have low-grade manifestations[16]. Affective exacerbations are invariably marked by psychosocial impairment, which may range from mild to severe. During the inter-episode, patients may manifest a varying degree of difficulties in day-to-day functioning and have problems in social, occupational and academic areas.

Major Depressive Disorder with Psychotic Features

MDD can be mild, moderate or severe depending on the relentless nature of symptoms and their impact on the day-to-day performance of the patient. Although psychotic features like delusions and hallucinations are not part of the core criteria, these may be present in moderate to severe MDD. The psychotic manifestations are often mood congruent and reflective of the depressed affective tone, but can also be mood incongruent and include such symptoms as paranoid delusions, ideas of reference, hypochondriacal and somatic delusions and hallucinations. In the latter event, the depressive nature of the illness may be difficult to recognize and the disease may be indistinguishable from schizoaffective disorder which is considered a psychotic spectrum condition.[17] With the current state of knowledge it can be surmised that MDD patients with psychotic symptoms tend to have prolonged episodes without significant periods of remission and their course and prognosis is more akin to people with schizophrenia spectrum disorders.[18]

Melancholic Depression

An important subtype of the disorder is MDD with melancholic features. In this condition there is a distinct flavor to the depressed mood, characterized by anhedonia or loss of pleasure in day-to-day activities. There is marked diurnal variation as the patient feels worse during the morning with varying degrees of improvement towards the latter afternoon and evening. There is severe insomnia, markedly reduced sleep duration and early morning wakening. Anorexia can be extreme with significant weight loss over a short period of time. Patients experience severe guilt which is often delusional in intensity, worthlessness, helplessness, hopelessness and suicidal ideation. Behavior is characterized by restlessness and psychomotor agitation. It can be construed that MDD with melancholic features is a particularly severe form of the disorder and is accompanied with discernible impairment in daily functioning. An interesting subtype is MDD with atypical features which is exemplified by reversed vegetative signs, that is, increased sleep and appetite with weight gain. While the mood is low, depression is usually mild to moderate, there is no diurnal mood variation or anhedonia. Patients have psychomotor retardation, and experience heaviness in the body, sometimes described as "leaden paralysis". Depression with atypical features may be comorbid with eating disorders such as bulimia nervosa and binge eating disorder, sleep disorders like obstructive sleep apnea and substance use disorders, particularly alcohol abuse.[19]

Bipolar Disorder

BD is considered a severe psychiatric illness, a type of mood disorder in which genetic polymorphisms play an overarching role; the diathesis runs in families, with several members being afflicted to varying degrees. It has two opposing modes of presentation, either as MDEs or manic/hypomanic exacerbations. Up to 40% of afflicted individuals may have simultaneous manifestations of both types, when the specifier "with mixed features" is applied to describe the mood episode. The disorder usually has an earlier age of onset than MDD and affects males and females equally. It is a chronic illness and follows a relapsing and remitting course throughout life. The treatment is primarily with mood stabilizers and all the current medications provide only symptomatic relief, rather than resulting in a complete cure. Due to complex and refractory presentations, treatment with multiple psychotropic agents is prevalent, referred to as "polypharmacy". This strategy often results in adverse effects, which is one factor in treatment of noncompliance from patients. Poorly managed BD whether from misdiagnosis, inappropriate treatment or patient noncompliance contributes to persistence of affective symptoms with adverse consequences in the biopsychosocial realms of functioning.[20] The ailment carries one the highest suicide rates among all psychiatric disorders and up to 50% of patients have a history of suicide attempts, with more than 10% succeeding in completing the act.[21]

Rapid Cycling

In this form of the disorder, BD patients have four or more affective episodes in a one year period. These exacerbations can be depressive, manic/hypomanic and may be accompanied with mixed features. It implies that the patient is rarely symptom free, as mood episodes recur either after a brief or essentially no period of remission. Rapid cycling is a particularly severe form of the disorder, afflicts around 30 to 40% of patients and is indicative of a poor prognosis. There may be a preponderance of females with rapid cycling, onset is in adolescence or early adulthood and the condition is frequently comorbid with other neuropsychiatric conditions, including anxiety spectrum disorders. Episodes can be of either polarity, but recurrent depressive episodes are, on the whole, more frequent, and may have a variable number of manic symptoms mixed in, leading to the specifier "depressive episode with mixed features". Because of episode severity psychotic manifestations are usually attendant, which can be both mood congruent or incongruent. In the latter instance the illness may be indistinguishable from schizoaffective disorder and merge into psychotic spectrum disorders. Anxiety disorders, particularly panic disorder, often coexists in rapid cycling patients and the presence of an increased number of anxiety symptoms aggravates the clinical picture. Furthermore, lack of impulse control leads to substance misuse, sexually promiscuous behavior and acts of aggression directed against self or others. Rapid cycling patients are prone to repeated acts of self-harm which can carry high potential for lethal consequence. There is also evidence this condition is poorly responsive to pharmacotherapy, so that the intractable nature of symptoms makes management a particularly challenging task.[22]

Somatic and Neuropsychiatric Comorbidities

The very high prevalence of medical, neurologic and psychiatric comorbid conditions with BD has led to the premise that this is actually a general bodily ailment affecting multiple systems and resulting in numerous manifestations. As such, the physician in charge must take a holistic view, and look for and preemptively treat conditions that are known to co-occur with this disease. Cohort association studies have demonstrated that metabolic abnormalities are a common accompaniment of BD. Glucose intolerance, pre-diabetes and diabetes mellitus often coexist in BD patients. Likewise, raised body mass index, increased waist circumference and frank obesity are prevalent in BD and recognized as endophenotypes of this condition. Dyslipidemia, low high density lipoprotein (HDL) to low density lipoprotein (LDL) ratio and high total cholesterol predispose to atherosclerosis and coronary artery disease and lead to premature mortality from cardiovascular conditions.[23] Many drugs used in the treatment of BD, in particular atypical antipsychotics, aggravate the metabolic syndrome and further complicate the management of these patients. The psychiatrist must be cognizant of such facts and pay special attention to these aspects for better patient outcomes.

Several neurological conditions are frequently found to co-occur with BD. Chief among these are migraine, fibromyalgia, idiopathic neuropathic pain, restless legs syndrome, vertigo and dizziness. Several medications used in the treatment of BD also have approved indications for these disorders. For example, topiramate is a United States Food and Drug Administration endorsed drug for migraine, gabapentin and pregabalin are licensed for neuropathic pain and restless legs syndrome, while other anticonvulsants such as lamotrigine and levetiracetam are also used for the same indications. These facts allude to shared mechanistic underpinnings of the said disorders and ongoing research may unravel the pathophysiologic substrates in this regard.[24] Finally, many psychiatric conditions are comorbid with BD and in this respect the treating physician must be especially cognizant of anxiety spectrum disorders, substance use disorders, eating disorders and posttraumatic stress disorder. Figure 1.3 gives an illustrative depiction of the clinical, psychological and physical sequelae arising from affective disturbances in BD.

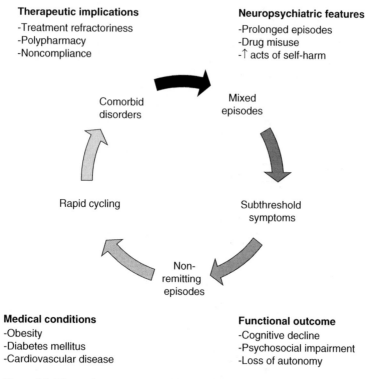

Therapeutic implications
-Treatment refractoriness
-Polypharmacy
-Noncompliance

Neuropsychiatric features
-Prolonged episodes
-Drug misuse
-↑ acts of self-harm

Comorbid
disorders

Mixed
episodes

Rapid cycling

Subthreshold
symptoms

Non-
remitting
episodes

Medical conditions
-Obesity
-Diabetes mellitus
-Cardiovascular disease

Functional outcome
-Cognitive decline
-Psychosocial impairment
-Loss of autonomy

Figure 1.3 The malignant course of bipolar disorder and its biopsychosocial
consequences

In the majority of patients with BD, the course of the disease is characterized by progressive worsening. This is represented by neuroprogression, cognitive decline, physical comorbidities and functional impairment. Persistent affective state has a pervasive negative effect on all physiological functions and progression of the diathesis results in adverse health consequences for every system of the body.

Seasonal Affective Disorder

Seasonal affective disorder (SAD) is a specific form of mood disorder since it follows a seasonal pattern and is associated with recurrent MDEs in autumn and winter months, which tend to remit in spring and summer. In the case of BD, MDEs may be followed by manic or hypomanic periods in the long daylight months of the summer equinox. An estimated 5% of the population is affected by SAD, and this incidence increases with residence in the northern latitudes.[25] It is conceivable that a number of physiological disturbances are responsible for SAD, such as diurnal rhythm instability epitomized by the phase shift hypothesis, which is regarded as the main abnormality in the extant literature.[26] Further causal mechanisms could comprise retinal sensitivity to light, neurotransmitter imbalance (norepinephrine, dopamine, acetylcholine), single nucleotide polymorphisms affecting circadian genes

Table 1.2 Clinical features of Seasonal Affective Disorder (SAD) according to DSM-5

- SAD is presently categorized under MDD, in addition to BD type I or II disorder.
- The affective disturbance is considered to have a seasonal pattern when there is reoccurrence of MDE at a specific period of the calendar year, usually autumn and winter.
- If there are repeated stressors that precipitate an MDE in a seasonal manner, then the "seasonal pattern specifier" does not apply.
- In the case of remission of the MDE, this must happen at a definite time of the year. Also change of polarity to mania/hypomania must also follow a seasonal pattern.
- In order to fulfill the "seasonal specifier" criteria two consecutive episodes of major depression must occur in two successive years.
- Non-seasonal episodes of major depression should not have taken place during the period of seasonal episodes.
- MDE with seasonal occurrence should occur more often than the non-season related MDE over the course of the patient's disease history.

BD – bipolar disorder; MDD – major depressive disorder; MDE – major depressive episode

and alterations of the serotonin transporter protein.[27] The current hypothesis assumes SAD is likely considered a multifaceted condition arising from several paths, each of which has individual involvement in the pathophysiology of the diathesis.

When SAD is considered the underlying diagnosis, the clinician must give credence to the condition if the mood episodes have a seasonal occurrence with recurring MDEs in the fall and winter, followed by euthymia or change of polarity to mania or hypomania in summer. The reappearance of this temporal representation twice in two consecutive years qualifies for the specifier "with seasonal pattern" to be applied to MDD or BD. Table 1.2 gives the clinical features of this condition according to DSM-5.

A review of the pertinent literature reveals that bright light therapy, antidepressants, in particular selective serotonic reuptake inhibitors (SSRIs), and cognitive behavioral therapy are suitable treatment options, and can be applied individually or in combination.[28] In the instance of bright light therapy the patients are placed about 1 to 1.5 feet from a white, luminous, well-lit equipment delivery system that provides light at a typical measure of 10,000 lux for half an hour each day just after sunrise. The subjects must have their eyes open; however they are not supposed to gaze directly into the light, since as long as the light enters the pupils the treatment is acceptable. Clinically significant improvement is often seen after the first few weeks of light treatment; nonetheless early cessation can lead to relapse and ideally the therapy needs to be carried on until the onset of natural decrease in symptoms in springtime or the beginning of mid-summer. In order to prevent a later episode, subjects may begin light therapy in the early fall when symptoms tend to reappear.[29] The purported mechanism of early morning bright light therapy is a robust phase advance and realignment of the circadian rhythm. Nonetheless, there is a caveat as BD patients can switch into mania or hypomania, have mixed states or rapid cycling. In conclusion, the presentation of seasonal pattern in major mood disorders is reminiscent of the fact that the circadian cycle is fundamentally disturbed and all effective treatments essentially resynchronize the circadian clock.

Conclusion

Here an endeavor has been made to outline the most pertinent aspects of major mood disorders. The current nosological classifications do not differentiate between MDD and BD as far as the diagnostic criteria for a MDE are concerned. However, these are discrete conditions with etiopathologic differences, distinct management protocols and disparate prognostic implications. When treating a patient with a major mood disorder, the practitioner must be alert for masquerading bipolarity in the case of MDD. Furthermore, the systemic nature of these conditions must be kept in mind and particular attention should be given to general medical comorbidities. In this regard, the clinician must perform regular physical examinations, obtain pertinent laboratory parameters and be always on the lookout for metabolic and other abnormalities. Since no curative treatments are available for major mood disorders, physicians should use clinical judgment in managing their patients on a day-to-day basis and employ the biopsychosocial model to achieve the best results.

Summary Points

- Major mood disorders are exemplified by MDD and BD.
- MDD is typified by unipolar depression and recurrent MDEs characterize the disorder.
- The occurrence of a single manic or hypomanic episode in MDD changes the diagnosis to bipolar disorder.
- The usual time of onset is in early adulthood and these ailments follow a relapsing and remitting course throughout life.
- There are numerous adverse consequences of mood disorders in the biopsychosocial spheres of functioning.
- Current understanding dictates these are systemic conditions that afflict all organ systems of the body.
- Management of mood disorders is challenging and existing treatments are, in essence, symptomatic rather than having a fully restorative value.

References

1) Hippius H, Müller N. The work of Emil Kraepelin and his research group in München. Eur Arch Psychiatry Clin Neurosci 2008;258 Suppl 2:3–11.
2) Kessler RC, Petukhova M, Sampson NA, Zaslavsky AM, Wittchen HU. Twelve-month and lifetime prevalence and lifetime risk of anxiety and mood disorders in the United States. Int J Methods Psychiatr Res 2012;21(3):169–184.

3) Peselow ED, Naghdechi L, Pizano D, IsHak WW. Polypharmacy in maintenance of bipolar disorder. Clin Neuropharmacol 2016;39:132–4.

4) Mansur RB, Brietzke E, McIntyre RS. Is there a "metabolic-mood syndrome"? A review of the relationship between obesity and mood disorders 2015. Neurosci Biobehav Rev 2015;52:89–104.

5) Phillips JA. A changing epidemiology of suicide? The influence of birth cohorts on suicide rates in the United States. Soc Sci Med 2014;114:151–160.

6) Lecrubier Y. Widespread underrecognition and undertreatment of anxiety and mood disorders: results from 3 European studies. J Clin Psychiatry 2007;68 Suppl 2:36–41.

7) Vohringer PA, Perlis RH. Discriminating between bipolar disorder and major depressive disorder. Psychiatr Clin North Am 2016;39:1–10.

8) Park SC, Sakong J, Koo BH, Kim JM, Jun TY, Lee MS, et al. Clinical significance of the number of depressive symptoms in major depressive disorder: results from the CRESEND study. J Korean Med Sci 2016;31:617–622.

9) Lorenzo-Luaces L. Heterogeneity in the prognosis of major depression: from the common cold to a highly debilitating and recurrent illness. Epidemiol Psychiatr Sci 2015;24:466–472.

10) Gignac A, McGirr A, Lam RW, Yatham LN. Recovery and recurrence following a first episode mania: a systematic review and meta-analysis of prospectively characterized cohorts. J Clin Psychiatry 2015;76:1241–1248.

11) Parker GB, Graham RK. An evaluation of the DSM-5 rules defining mania and hypomania with identical symptom criteria. J Affect Disord 2015;170:91–94.

12) Takeshima M, Oka T. DSM-5 defined 'mixed features' and Bennazi's mixed depression: which is practically useful to discriminate bipolar disorder from unipolar depression in patients with depression? Psychiatry Clin Neurosci 2015;69:109–116.

13) Shim IH, Woo YS, Bahk WM. Prevalence rates and clinical implications of bipolar disorder "with mixed features" as defined by DSM-5. J Affect Disord 2015;173:120–125.

14) McElroy SL, Keck PE Jr. Metabolic syndrome in bipolar disorder: a review with a focus on bipolar depression. J Clin Psychiatry 2014;75:46–61.

15) Muneer A. Staging models in bipolar disorder: a systematic review of the literature. Clin Psychopharmacol Neurosci 2016;14:117–130.

16) Mcintyre RS, Lee Y, Mansur RB. Treating to target in major depressive disorder: response to remission to functional recovery. CNS Spectr 2015;20 Suppl 1:20–30.

17) Rink L, Pagel T, Franklin J, Baethge C. Characteristics and heterogeneity of schizoaffective disorder compared with unipolar depression and schizophrenia – a systematic literature review and meta-analysis. J Affect Disord 2016;191:8–14.

18) Tohen M, Khalsa HM, Salvatore P, Vieta E, Ravichandran C, Baldessarini RJ. Two-year outcomes in first-episode psychotic depression: the McLean-Harvard First-Episode Project. J Affect Disord 2012;136:1–8.

19) Sculthorpe LD, Douglass AB. Sleep pathologies in depression and the clinical utility of polysomnography. Can J Psychiatry 2010;55:413–421.

20) Fornaro M, De Berardis D, Koshy AS, Perna G, Valchera A, Vancampfort D, et al. Prevalence and clinical features associated with bipolar disorder polypharmacy: a systematic review. Neuropsychiatr Dis Treat 2016;12:719–735.

21) Dennehy EB, Marangell LB, Allen MH, Chessick C, Wisnieswski SR, Thase ME. Suicide and suicide attempts in Systematic Treatment Enhancement Program for Bipolar Disorder (STEP-BD) 2011. J Affect Disord;133:423–427.

22) Carvalho AF, Dimellis D, Gonda X, Vieta E, McIntyre RS, Fountoulakis KN. Rapid cycling in bipolar disorder: a systematic review. J Clin Psychiatry 2014;75:e578–86.

23) Godin O, Etain B, Henry C, Bougerol T, Courtet P, Mayliss L, et al. Metabolic syndrome in a French cohort of patients with bipolar disorder: results from the FACE-BD cohort. J Clin Psychiatry 2014;75:1078–1085.

24) Bialer M. Why are antiepileptic drugs used for nonepileptic conditions? Epilepsia 2012;53 Suppl 7:26–33.

25) Kurlansik SL, Ibay AD. Seasonal affective disorder. Am Fam Physician 2012;86(11):1037–1041.

26) Nagy AD, Iwamoto A, Kawai M, Goda R, Matsuo H, Otsuka T, et al. Melatonin adjusts the expression pattern of clock genes in the supraschiasmatic nucleus and induces antidepressant-like effect in a mouse model of seasonal affective disorder. Chronobiol Int 2015;32:447–457.

27) Mc Mahon B, Andersen SB, Madsen MK, Hjordt LV, Hageman I, Dam H, et al. Seasonal difference in brain serotonin transporter binding predicts symptom severity in patients with seasonal affective disorder. Brain 2016;189:1605–1614.

28) Danilenko KV, Ivanova IA. Dawn stimulation versus bright light in seasonal affective disorder: treatment effects and subjective preference. J Affect Disord 2015;180:87–89.

29) Nussbaumer B, Kaminski-Hartenthaler A, Forneris CA, Morgan LC, Sonis JH, Gaynes BN, et al. Light therapy for preventing seasonal affective disorder. Chochrane Database Syst Rev 2015;(11):CD011269.

2 Major Mood Disorders
Differentiating Features

Introduction

Major mood disorders, including major depressive disorder (MDD) and bipolar disorder (BD), are among the most common psychiatric conditions. In a relatively recent international survey of 18 countries the average lifetime prevalence of major depressive episodes (MDEs) was 14.6% in ten high income countries and 11.1% in eight low-to-middle income nations.[1] The population studied was not stratified according to the type of mood disorder, so it can be assumed that the patients comprised of both MDD and BD as long as they fulfilled the Diagnostic and Statistical Manual of Mental Disorders – 4th Edition (DSM-IV) criteria for a MDE. The current nosological classifications (International Classification of Diseases – 10th Revision [ICD-10] and the Diagnostic and Statistical Manual of Mental Disorders – 5th Edition [DSM-5]) do not distinguish between these disorders in so far as the diagnostic features of depression are concerned, but MDD and BD have fundamental neurobiological differences with therapeutic and prognostic implications. These are dissimilar conditions, with polymorphisms in disparate genes causing biological alterations that result in distinct phenotypes. Consequentially, there are dissimilar presentations, and diverging illness trajectories that require implementation of discrete management plans.[2] Such emerging insights are reflected in the DSM-5 in which a necessary shift has been implemented by segregating the two conditions into separate chapters, whereas previously these were described under the common rubric of "mood disorders".

Allostatic Load Model of Mood Disorders

Mood disorders are complex gene x environment diseases and are heterogeneous in symptomatic expression. Current knowledge assumes these disorders lie on a spectrum with depression and mania being opposite poles of the mood disturbance that has myriad presentations, confounded by such factors as personality characteristics, neuropsychiatric comorbidities and psychosocial incumbencies.[3] In the early phase of mood disorders, stress factors are

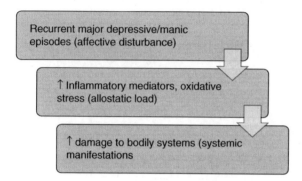

Figure 2.1 Linking biological and clinical findings to affective disturbances in mood disorders

Biological findings	Clinical findings
– ↑↑pro-inflammatory cytokines	– ↑episode severity
– ↓anti-inflammatory cytokines	– ↑episode frequency
– ↓neurotrophic support	– ↑suicidality
– ↑oxidative stress	– ↓cognitive functioning
– ↑apoptosis of neurons	– ↓functioning in daily affairs

identified as precipitating events, but with the advancement of the diathesis affective episodes recur spontaneously. Additionally, asymptomatic periods become progressively shorter and an unrelenting disease state ensues which causes impairments in cognitive and functional domains.[4] At the latter stages the clinical picture is characterized by rapid cycling, residual affective states and subthreshold symptoms. The overall consequence is "neuroprogression" which is epitomized by a decline in autonomy, and impairment of role functioning with a resulting loss of personal independence.[5] Therefore, the advanced stages of mood disorders are typified by severe psychosocial and biological disturbances, with incremental damage to central and peripheral systems of the body as a consequence of increased "allostatic load".[6] This is mediated by such biological factors as a persistent proinflammatory state, increased oxidative stress, decreased neurotrophic support and apoptosis of neurons in key mood regulating areas of the brain. Figure 2.1 gives a schematic representation of the allostatic load model of mood disorders.

Mood Disorders as Systemic Ailments

Mood disorders impose an immense burden in the biopsychosocial domains. Patients are initially affected in youth or early adulthood and have relapses and recurrences throughout their lifetimes. These are in essence, multisystem disorders affecting essentially the entire body and leading to increased morbidity and mortality from such conditions as diabetes mellitus, adiposity, metabolic disturbances and cardiovascular diseases.[7] The mechanisms through which so many bodily systems are adversely affected are incompletely understood and the current available treatments do not target the core abnormalities. Because of less than optimal therapeutic measures, patients continue to experience neuropsychiatric symptoms and incur ongoing damage to different organ systems, so that the overall prognosis is unsatisfactory.[8] In this scenario, for the sake of effective patient management it is crucial to develop a better understanding of major mood disorders. Clinically, the depressive phase of MDD and BD is alike, but certain disease characteristics can be helpful in differentiating the two conditions and these are discussed next.

Differentiating Features of Unipolar and Bipolar Depression

Disease Onset

The *sine qua non* of BD is a manic episode, but in practice depression is its most frequent presentation.[9] Longitudinal naturalistic studies show that bipolar patients spend the majority of their time in the depressed state, rather than being manic or hypomanic.[10] The former can manifest as MDEs, or as subthreshold symptoms. Additionally, depressive manifestations can intermingle with manic or hypomanic symptoms and give rise to mixed states, which portend a worse clinical outcome.[11] Whereas in unipolar depression the first episode occurs around the mid-20s, bipolar depression has a much earlier onset, in early teenage years. Moreover, it is often the index mood episode in BD and has melancholic features[12]. This disorder is notorious in masquerading in innumerable forms and the presenting illness can be in the form of anxiety spectrum disorders, conduct disorders and substance use disorders. Because of these reasons BD is misidentified and the lag period in diagnosis is of the magnitude of several years.[13]

Unipolar Versus Bipolar Depression

The major depressive episodes in MDD can be single or recurrent, but tend to be discrete with well-characterized periods of remission. In the case of BD, patients are symptomatic for longer periods; they may have severe mood episodes or sub-syndromal symptoms in the inter-episode. Rapid cycling is a phenomenon in which BD patients have four or more affective episodes in a 12-month period. This is regarded as an extreme form of the disorder with adverse consequences in the functional and psychological domains.[14] With repeated mood episodes there is neuroprogression and deterioration in all aspects of living, which in essence implies the persistence of a deficit state with eventual loss of self-independence.[15] The suicide rate is very high in BD and this may be attributable to many factors, chief among which are greater number and severity of episodes, existence of mixed states and the presence of such comorbidities as anxiety spectrum and substance use disorders.[16]

In this scenario, when a patient presents with a major depressive episode, the primary question for the treating physician is the correct identification of the mood disorder. Although there are no validated criteria for such a distinction, certain features should alert the clinician. This is important because treatment of BD is primarily with mood stabilizers, whereas unipolar depression is best managed with standard antidepressant medications.[17] Administration of antidepressants without adjunctive mood stabilizers to BD patients can result in manic/hypomanic switches, induction of mixed states and rapid cycling.[18]

Illness Characteristics

When a patient first presents with a depressive episode, the presence of family history of BD is a cautionary sign. Age of onset is significant, as the index episode in BD occurs during adolescence or teenage years, while this is usually later in major depression. Furthermore, as BD patients tend to have recurrent, severe mood episodes they often have a history of psychiatric hospitalizations.[19] Major depression that is treatment resistant to two or more first-line antidepressant medications should raise the suspicion of a covert bipolar diathesis. Unipolar patients who shift to mania or hypomania when treated with antidepressants, electroconvulsive therapy (ECT) or chronobiological measures are considered to lie on the bipolar spectrum. In this regard, seasonal variation may be marked in BD with patients experiencing repeated depressive episodes during fall and winter months.[20]

With respect to clinical presentation, patients with bipolar depression often experience mixed features such as racing thoughts, irritability, grandiose ideation and increased energy. Moreover, they are prone to having recurrent suicidal ideation, and a history of repeated self-injurious behavior in unipolar depression should indicate an underlying bipolar illness.[21] Neuropsychiatric and physical comorbidities are frequently associated with BD including panic disorder, posttraumatic stress disorder, substance use disorders, borderline personality disorder and eating disorders.[22] Neurological conditions found more often in bipolar patients include migraine, idiopathic neuropathic pain, vertigo and restless legs syndrome.[23] An important caveat with respect to the bipolar diathesis is its association with the metabolic syndrome, obesity and diabetes mellitus, so that cardiovascular diseases are the foremost cause of premature mortality in this group of people.[24] In conclusion, it can be construed that among mood disorders, BD is a more severe condition and the clinician must be vigilant not to misdiagnose it. Table 2.1 gives a summary of the clinical features that should alert clinicians for the possible presence of bipolar spectrum disorders in patients presenting with major depressive episodes.

Table 2.1 Likely indicators of bipolarity in patients presenting with major depressive episodes

1) Onset in adolescence or early teenage years
2) Family history of bipolar disorder
3) Comorbid anxiety, substance use or conduct disorders
4) Major depressive episode with melancholic features
5) Psychotic depression
6) Repeated mood episodes
7) Increased severity of episodes, with history of hospitalization
8) Treatment-resistant depression
9) Mixed states
10) Seasonal affective disorder
11) Suicidal behavior/repeated attempts at self-harm
12) Switching on antidepressants

Affective Ailments as Spectrum Disorders

The Continuum of Mood Disturbances

Fluctuations in mood are commonly experienced by people, particularly when they face stressful life events. Nevertheless, if mood swings are prominent and persistent and result in notable distress or impairment, there could be an underlying mood disorder. The latter can be classified along a spectrum defined by the extent and severity of mood elevation, from unipolar depression to bipolar type II to bipolar type I disorders.[25] Individuals with unipolar depression present with depressive episodes only, and those with bipolar II or I disorder exhibit progressively more obvious periods of sustained mood elevation from hypomania to well-characterized mania. This continuum of affective disturbances is thoroughly understood and reflected in the current versions of diagnostic classifications. Figure 2.2 provides an illustrative adaptation of the modern version of mood disorders as spectrum conditions.

Epidemiological Considerations

Bipolar spectrum disorders affect approximately 4% of the world's population irrespective of nationality, ethnic origin or socioeconomic status and represent one of the leading causes of disability.[26] In the case of MDD, the estimated lifetime prevalence is higher in different surveys, of the order of 14%. As regards sex, bipolar I disorder affects men and women equally, whereas bipolar II disorder is more common in women. With respect to MDD, women predominate over men.

Mood Disorders in Low Income Countries

There is an acute dearth of mental health services in low income countries, access to psychiatric care is limited and scarce provisions imply the management

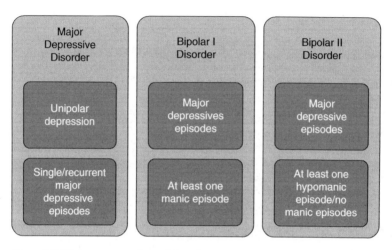

Figure 2.2 The spectrum of mood disorders

Major mood disorders are exemplified by major depressive disorder, which is characterized by a single or recurrent episode of unipolar depression, bipolar disorder type I, which has repeated depressive and manic episodes, and bipolar disorder type II, marked by depressive and hypomanic episodes only.

of mood disorders is particularly challenging in resource-poor nations. In this respect, the overall spending on public health comprises a very small fraction of the total expenditure, and in many countries either no allocations are made for mental health or this amount is negligible. Consequentially, patients with psychiatric ailments essentially receive no help with acute management or ongoing psychosocial care. There is a critical shortage of trained staff, including psychiatrists, psychologists and mental health nurses all of which adversely affects the care of psychiatric patients in general and mood disorder patients in particular. The feeble infrastructure of mental health services provides further difficulty for psychiatric patients and has a negative impact on the society as a whole, with entire families feeling left out. It is imperative that problems faced by mentally ill patients are properly projected, so that governments of less developed nations pay attention to the plight of this section of the society, since in the absence of this understanding progress cannot be made.

Diagnostic Implications

Previously known as manic depressive insanity, BD is a severe, chronic mood disorder characterized by manic, mixed or depressive episodes. While there is no fixed pattern of episode recurrence, many patients exhibit a typical polarity of illness with manic or depressive preponderance of affective exacerbations.[27] No biomarker has been validated for any mood disorder, which implies that diagnosis is established on clinical criteria and is entirely empirically based.

Table 2.2 The diagnosis of bipolar disorder and related conditions according to DSM-5

■ **BD type I:**
The occurrence of at a minimum one manic episode, while MDEs are usual but not required for diagnosis.

■ **BD type II:**
There must be the presence of at a minimum one hypomanic episode and one MDE.

■ **Cyclothymic disorder:**
Recurrent hypomanic and depressive exacerbations for a continued period of two years, the latter not fulfilling the criteria for MDEs.

■ **Correlated mood disorders:**
Affective disturbances which do not fulfill the diagnostic requirements for BD type I, BD type II or cyclothymic disorder due to inadequate time interval or fewer number of symptoms, for example:
 • Hypomanic episodes which last less than 4 days along with MDE
 • Hypomanic periods with only a few symptoms and MDE
 • A condition in which a hypomanic episode occurs in the absence of MDE
 • Cyclothymic disorder which is less than 2 years duration

■ **Bipolar disorder NOS:**
A residual category in which affective manifestations are present but do not fulfill diagnostic requirements of a specific disorder.

■ **Substance-induced condition:**
BD provoked by an illicit substance or medication.

■ **BD caused by a general medical condition:**
BD caused by a medical or neurological disorder.

BD – bipolar disorder; MDE – major depressive episode; NOS – not otherwise specified

The most widely acknowledged diagnostic classifications are the International Classification of Diseases – 10th Revision (ICD-10) and the Diagnostic and Statistical Manual of Mental Disorders – 5th Edition (DSM-5). Mood disorders are recognized by the longitudinal course which is marked by acute flare ups, as well as subthreshold symptoms.[28] Due to the presence of manic episodes bipolar I disorder might seem to have a more tortuous evolution and worse prognosis than bipolar II disorder; however, the latter is characterized by high episode frequency, soaring rates of psychiatric comorbidities and recurrent suicidal behaviors that makes it a very disabling condition.[29] The bipolar spectrum encompasses several disorders and Table 2.2 gives an outline of the various conditions included under this rubric. In contrast, MDD is typified by recurrent depressive episodes, discrete affective exacerbations and more complete periods of remission. There are lower rates of comorbidities and a benign illness course is evident in a significant number of patients.

Illness Trajectory

The natural history of mood disorders includes periods of remission, but recurrence is the norm, particularly if adherence to treatment is poor. In BD, the polarity of the index episode can predict the polarity of subsequent episodes. Patients with a depressive predominant polarity often have a depressive onset, history of suicide attempts, and a likely seasonal pattern; they often carry the diagnosis of bipolar II disorder.[30] Conversely, with a manic predominant polarity onset is in youth, drug misuse and disturbances of conduct are frequent and patients receive the diagnosis of bipolar I disorder.[31] Bipolar spectrum disorders are often comorbid with anxiety disorders and psychotic symptoms may also occur, in which case differentiation from schizoaffective disorder may become difficult. The illness can be treatment refractory and in many patients there is progressive decline in functioning in the biopsychosocial domains. In MDD, the course is relapsing and remitting and there may be complete periods of recovery between episodes. Rates of psychiatric and medical comorbidities are lower, individual functioning is preserved and the majority of patients do not progress to the later stages.

Suicide in Mood Disorders

People with mood disorders are at very high risk of death by suicide. The incidence of death by suicide among patients with BD is elevated, and can be more than 20 times higher than in the general population, particularly when BD is inadequately treated. About a third to a half of patients with BD attempt suicide at least once in their lifetime, and roughly 15–20% of the attempts are completed. Variables significantly associated with suicide attempts include female sex, young age at onset of illness, depressive polarity of illness, comorbid anxiety and substance abuse disorders and borderline personality disorder. By contrast, factors frequently linked with death by suicide include male sex, family history of suicide, violent method of self-harm and high degree of intent and secrecy.[32] Correspondingly, in MDD many patients experience suicidal ideation and with increasing severity of illness the risk of completed suicide becomes higher. The occurrence of mixed symptoms in MDD patients greatly elevates the threat for suicidal behavior. The presence of anxiety and substance abuse are other contributing factors. In this regard, it must be appreciated that mood disorder patients who have medical diseases, for example ischemic heart disease, rheumatoid arthritis or other inflammatory conditions are prone to suicidal behavior. Prompt and comprehensive assessment and management of suicidal ideation in patients with mood disorders is of great importance. Appraisal of risk should include the intention to commit suicide, availability and potential lethality of methods and the presence of psychiatric and medical comorbidities. Finally, such protective factors as family and social support should also be taken into account in the overall assessment.

Psychometric Scales

Hypomania is an under-recognized mood state but is, nonetheless, common. Patients do not always recall or read their mood accurately nor judge its consequences, and sometimes enjoy the mood state and view it as desirable. However, hypomania often heralds a manic or depressive episode, with ensuing severe consequences. Although patients typically struggle with depression, families and close associates often complain about the problematic outcomes of hypomanic episodes. Thus, the clinician must be on the lookout for hypomanic symptoms and should not let subtle changes in mood go unrecognized. In the clinical setting both history and mental state examination are helpful in this regard. However, a psychometric scale with good specificity and sensitivity can be invaluable and provides a measure of objectivity to the diagnostic process. In day-to-day practice, an instrument with such attributes is the Hypomania Checklist 32 (HCL-32), which is employed for the screening of hypomanic symptoms in patients with major depression.[33] Easily administered, HCL-32 is helpful in diagnosing bipolarity in MDD subjects who experience subclinical symptoms and have never experienced full-fledged manic episodes. There is a caveat, all elements of assessment such as longitudinal course, family history and treatment response must be taken into account to correctly diagnose a depressed patient with bipolar spectrum disorders. Once a diagnosis of hypomania is made, other scales such as the Young Mania Rating Scale can be used to assess the severity of mood elevation.

The DSM-5 criteria for major depressive episode are the same for BD and unipolar depression. The severity of the major depressive episode can be assessed with the help of validated instruments, the most commonly used being the Hamilton Rating Scale for Depression (HRSD) and the Montgomery-Asberg Depression Rating Scale (MADRS). The main divergence between the two scales is that MADRS is more sensitive to changes in affective symptomatology; it may not place as much emphasis on somatic manifestations of depression as does the HRSD. Otherwise both measures are highly authenticated and frequently utilized in clinical practice, as well as research.

Differentiating Between Unipolar and Bipolar Depression

The clinical differentiation between unipolar and bipolar depression has been a matter of concern for psychiatrists for many decades. In the 1950s, Leonhard was the first to describe differences between the two conditions and a decade later Angst, Perris, Winokur and colleagues further clarified these distinctions. Although there are no pathognomonic signs, these researchers described some clinical features that are useful in discriminating between the two conditions.[34] In this respect, the following aspects are noteworthy:

1) Bipolar depression has an earlier age of onset.
2) Depressive episodes in BD are more frequent and tend to be of shorter duration.
3) Bipolar depression has an abrupt onset and termination.
4) It is often associated with comorbid substance abuse.

5) Bipolar depression frequently co-occurs with panic and other anxiety disorders.
6) It is triggered by stressors during the early stages.
7) It is often post-partum in onset.
8) Atypical symptoms, such as hypersomnia, lability and weight instability are common in bipolar depression being reported in the majority of cases, but these are described in less than half of those with unipolar depression.
9) Psychosis, psychomotor retardation, and catatonia are more characteristic of bipolar depression.
10) Somatic complaints like aches and pains, fatigability and gastrointestinal symptoms are more frequent in unipolar depression.
11) Finally, family history of mania is an important indicator of bipolarity.

Catatonic Symptoms in Mood Disorders

Catatonia can be defined as a neurobehavioral syndrome that has motor, psychic and autonomic manifestations and can occur in a wide range of medical, neurological and psychiatric conditions. The etiology of this distinctive syndrome is not fully understood, but emerging evidence indicates that biological stress facilitated by inflammatory mediators and reactive oxygen species leads to imbalance of neurotransmitters in the brain and precipitates the catatonic state.[35] Catatonic symptoms can be present in any severe phase of major mood disorders, when the specifier "with catatonic features" is applied to describe the particular episode. There is a wide range of catatonic symptoms; behavioral manifestations can vary from negativism, withdrawal, staring, immobility/stupor, mutism, posturing, grimacing, stereotypies, and mannerisms to non-purposeful excitement, undirected combativeness, unexplained impulsive behavior, echopraxia and echolalia. Motor abnormalities can include rigidity, waxy flexibility (when moved passively the limbs maintain their position), catalepsy (the person sustains a certain posture irrespective of environmental changes), mitgehen (anglepoise lamp sign) and gegenhalten (involuntary variable resistance during passive movement). According to DSM-5, if two of the abovementioned signs are present then the specifier "with catatonic features" can be used. Evidence from the extant literature suggests patients with mood disorders are regularly afflicted with catatonia and this state can emerge in both MDD and BD.[36]

Some forms of catatonia can endanger life, for example the patient's refusal to eat or drink, extreme and unsustainable excitement, or the development of severe autonomic instability.[37] In both males and females catatonic features can complicate any severe affective episode and patients of any age can present with catatonic symptoms. As alluded to above, catatonic symptoms are well recognized to occur in numerous medical and neurological conditions, whereas in psychiatric practice these are most often encountered in schizophrenia and mood disorders. Catatonia has also been described in the literature as grafted on to autistic disorder. A particularly dangerous form of catatonia is associated with autonomic instability – hyperthermia, tachycardia, blood pressure variations and diaphoresis. This condition, termed malignant catatonia, is symptom-wise and is indistinguishable from neuroleptic malignant syndrome (NMS). In NMS, however, there is the history of exposure to an antipsychotic agent which is not so in the case of malignant catatonia.[38] Catatonic symptoms consistently and adequately respond to electroconvulsive therapy, which is therefore regarded as the first-line treatment.[39] Among medications, benzodiazepines have shown efficacy; in particular, lorazepam has been used both orally and intravenously to treat catatonic patients. While oral lorazepam has been associated with variable results, intravenous administration has been more successful. However, in patients responsive to lorazepam, continuous oral dosing or repeated intravenous administrations are required to suppress catatonic symptoms. As a final note, it can be construed that catatonia is a rather neglected complication of mood disorders; nevertheless clinicians must always be on the lookout for its presence, be cognizant of its consequences and should have the necessary knowledge to treat it appropriately.

Conclusion

MDD is characterized by unipolar depression, whereas BD is typified by the occurrence of at least one manic or hypomanic episode. Both diseases impose a very high burden on the patients and are challenging to manage, particularly in the context of scarce psychiatric provisions. This is particularly so in developing nations, where allocation of meagre resources to the mental health system adversely affects the outcome of affective illnesses, and increases the predicament of the patients and their families. To appropriately treat the two conditions, it is crucial to distinguish between them. In this chapter an attempt has been made to highlight those clinical features that are helpful in this regard. It is hoped that equipped with this knowledge, clinicians would be better able to manage their patients, with improved results for those afflicted by these intractable diseases.

Summary Points

- MDD is represented by unipolar depression, whereas BD is exemplified by the occurrence of at least one manic or hypomanic episode.
- Both diseases carry high morbidity and mortality, though for a variety of reasons BD appears to have a worse prognosis.
- Depressive episodes are essentially similar in the two conditions; however, certain features may be helpful in differentiating between major mood disorders.
- Major mood disorders are spectrum conditions and there is a high rate of conversion from unipolar depression to BD in the affected patients.

- When assessing a patient with a mood disorder, the clinician should adopt a meticulous approach, keep the differential diagnosis in mind and treat him or her empirically.
- To date there are no biomarkers to assist in diagnosis and management, so treatment is essentially based on clinical judgment, but certain psychometric scales can help in this regard.
- Finally, it is of note that patients with any severe affective disturbance can develop the catatonic syndrome which is often missed and goes untreated unless the clinician has a high level of alertness.

References

1) Bromet E, Andrade LH, Hwang I, Sampson NA, Alonso J, de Girolamo G, et al. Cross-national epidemiology of DSM-IV major depressive episode. BMC Med 2011;9:90.

2) Moreno C, Hasin DS, Arango C, Oquendo MA, Vieta E, Liu S, et al. Depression in bipolar disorder versus major depressive disorder: results from the National Epidemiologic Survey on Alcohol and Related Conditions. Bipolar Disord 2012;14:271–282.

3) Becker DF, Grilo CM. Comorbidity of mood and substance use disorders in patients with binge-eating disorder: associations with personality disorder and eating disorder pathology. J Psychosom Res 2015;79:159–164.

4) Moylan S, Maes M, Wray NR, Berk M. The neuroprogressive nature of major depressive disorder: pathways to disease evolution and resistance, and therapeutic implications. Mol Psychiatry 2013;18:595–606.

5) Vieta E, Reinares M, Rosa AR. Staging bipolar disorder. Neurotox Res 2011;19:279–285.

6) Kapczinski NS, Mwangi B, Cassidy RM, Librenza-Garcia D, Bermudez MB, Kauer-Sant'anna M, et al. Neuroprogression and illness trajectories in bipolar disorder. Expert Rev Neurother 2017;17:277–285.

7) Hajek T, McIntyre R, Alda M. Bipolar disorders, type 2 diabetes, and the brain. Curr Opin Psychiatry 2016;29:1–6.

8) Muneer A. The neurobiology of bipolar disorder: an integrated approach. Chonnam Med J 2016;52:18–37.

9) Miller S, Dell'Osso B, Ketter TA. The prevalence and burden of bipolar depression. J Affect Disord 2014;169 Suppl 1:S3–11.

10) De Dios C, Agud JL, Ezquiaga E, Garcia-Lopez A, Soler B, Vieta E. Syndromal and subsyndromal illness status and five year morbidity using criteria of the International Society of Bipolar Disorders compared to alternative criteria. Psychopathology 2012;45:102–108.

11) Valenti M, Pacchiarotti I, Undurraga J, Bonnin CM, Popovic D, Goikolea JM, et al. Risk factors for rapid cycling in bipolar disorder. Bipolar Disord 2015;17:549–559.

12) Bukh JD, Andersen PK, Kessing LV. Rates and predictors of remission, recurrence and conversion to bipolar disorder after the first lifetime episode of depression: a prospective 5-year follow-up study. Psychol Med 2016;46:1151–1161.

13) Nasrallah HA. Consequences of misdiagnosis: inaccurate treatment and poor patient outcomes in bipolar disorder. J Clin Psychiatry 2015;76:e1328.

14) Fountoulakis KN, Grunze H, Vieta E, Young A, Yatham L, Blier P, et al. The International College of Neuropsychopharmacology (CINP) treatment guidelines for bipolar disorder in adults (CINP-BD-2017), part 3: the clinical guidelines. Int J Neuropsychopharmacol 2017;20(2):180–195.

15) da Costa SC, Passos IC, Lowri C, Soares JC, Kapczinski F. Refractory bipolar disorder and neuroprogression. Prog Neuropsychopharmacol Biol Psychiatry 2016;70:103–110.

16) Rajewska-Rager A, Sibilski P, Lepczynska N. Risk factors for suicide among children and youths with bipolar spectrum and early bipolar disorder. Psychiatr Pol 2015;49:477–488.

17) Karanti A, Kardell M, Lundberg U, Landen M. Changes in mood stabilizer prescription patterns in bipolar disorder. J Affect Disord 2016;195:50–56.

18) Muneer A. Mixed states in bipolar disorder: etiology, pathogenesis and treatment. Chonnam Med J. 2017;53:1–13.

19) Shapiro J, Timmins V, Swampillai B, Scavone A, Collinger K, Boulos C, et al. Correlates of psychiatric hospitalization in a clinical sample of Canadian adolescents with bipolar disorder. Compr Psychiatry 2014;55:1855–1861.

20) Akhter A, Fiedorowicz JG, Zhang T, Potash JB, Cavanaugh J, Solomon DA, et al. Seasonal variation of manic and depressive symptoms in bipolar disorder. Bipolar Disord 2013;15:377–384.

21) Musliner KL, Munk-Olsen T, Laursen TM, Eaton WW, Zandi PP, Mortensen PB. Heterogeneity in 10-year course trajectories of moderate to severe major depressive disorder: a Danish national-register based study. JAMA Psychiatry 2016;73:346–353.

22) Simhandl C, Radua J, Konig B, Amann BL. Prevalence and impact of comorbid alcohol use disorder in bipolar disorder: a prospective follow-up study. Aust N Z J Psychiatry 2016;50:345–351.

23) Fornaro M, Stubbs B. A meta-analysis investigating the prevalence and moderators of migraines among people with bipolar disorder. J Affect Disord 2015;178:88–97.

24) Grover S, Nebhinani N, Chakrabarti S, Avasthi A, Basu D, Kulhara P, et al. Cardiovascular risk factors among bipolar disorder patients admitted to an inpatient unit of a tertiary care hospital in India. Asian J Psychiatr 2014;10:51–55.

25) Woo YS, Shim IH, Wang HR, Song HR, Jun TY, Bahk WM. A diagnosis of bipolar spectrum disorder predicts diagnostic conversion from unipolar depression to bipolar disorder: a 5-year retrospective study. J Affect Disord 2015;174:83–88.

26) Cerimele JM, Chwastiak LA, Dodson S, Katon WJ. The prevalence of bipolar disorder in general primary care samples: a systematic review. Gen Hosp Psychiatry 2014;36:19–25.

27) Carvalho AF, McIntyre RS, Dimelis D, Gonda X, Berk M, Nunes-Neto PR, et al. Predominant polarity as a course specifier for bipolar disorder: a systematic review. J Affect Disord 2014;163:56–64.

28) Gershon A, Eidelman P. Inter-episode affective intensity and instability: predictors of depression and functional impairment in bipolar disorder. J Behav Ther Exp Psychiatry 2015;46:14–18.

29) Goffin KC, Dell'Osso B, Miller S, Wang PW, Holtzman JN, Hooshmand F, et al. Different characteristics associated with suicide attempts among bipolar I versus bipolar II disorder patients. J Psychiatr Res 2016;76:94–100.

30) Tundo A, Musetti L, Benedetti A, Berti B, Massimetti G, Dell'Osso L. Onset polarity and illness course in bipolar I and bipolar II disorders: the predictive role of broadly defined mixed states. Compr Psychiatry 2015;63:15–21.

31) Popovic D, Torrent C, Goikolea JM, Cruz N, Sánchez-Moreno J, González-Pinto A, et al. Clinical implications of predominant polarity and the polarity index in bipolar disorder: a naturalistic study. Acta Psychiatr Scand 2014;129:366–374.

32) Costa Lda S, Alencar ÁP, Nascimento Neto PJ, dos Santos Mdo S, da Silva CG, Pinheiro Sde F, et al. Risk factors for suicide in bipolar disorder: a systematic review. J Affect Disord 2015;196:71–77.

33) Gamma A, Angst J, Azorin JM, Bowden CL, Perugi G, Vieta E, et al. Transcultural validity of the Hypomania Checklist-32 (HCL-32) in patients with major depressive episodes 2013. Bipolar Disord;15:701–712.

34) Hirschfeld RM. Differential diagnosis of bipolar disorder and major depressive disorder. J Affect Disord. 2014;169 Suppl 1:S12–16.

35) Gupta A, Kumar A, Kulkarni SK. Targeting oxidative stress, mitochondrial dysfunction and neuroinflammation signaling by selective cyclooxygenase (COX)-2 inhibitors mitigates MPTP-induced neurotoxicity in mice. Prog Neuropsychopharmacol Biol Psychiatry 2011;35:974–981.

36) Grover S, Chakrabarti S, Ghormode D, Agarwal M, Sharma A, Avasthi A. Catatonia in inpatients with psychiatric disorders: a comparison of schizophrenia and mood disorders. Psychiatry Res 2015;229(3):919–925.

37) Dessens FM, van Paassen J, van Westerloo DJ, van der Wee NJ, van Vliet IM, van Noorden MS. Electroconvulsive therapy in the intensive care unit for the treatment of catatonia: a case series and review of the literature. Gen Hosp Psychiatry 2016;38:37–41.

38) Lang FU, Lang S, Becker T, Jäger M. Neuroleptic malignant syndrome or catatonia? Trying to solve the catatonic dilemma. Psychopharmacology (Berl) 2015;232:1–5.

39) Ungvari GS. Catatonia in DSM-5: controversies regarding its psychopathology, clinical presentation and treatment response. Neuropsychopharmacol Hung 2014;16:189–194.

3   Comorbidity in Mood Disorders

Introduction

Mood disorders are associated with significant morbidity and mortality with an estimated reduction in life expectancy of 12–20 years for men and 11–17 years for women compared to the general population.[1] Although individuals with major depressive disorder (MDD) and bipolar disorder (BD) are at an increased risk of suicide, elevated rates of medical comorbidities (primarily cardiovascular disease) is believed to be the main reason for the observed decrease in life expectancy in major mood disorders.[2] Mortality secondary to cardiovascular diseases, diabetes mellitus, autoimmune disorders, chronic obstructive pulmonary disease and acute infections is higher in people with severe affective illnesses than the population in general.[3] For instance, cardiovascular disease is the leading cause of death in people with BD, with a significantly increased prevalence in comparison with both matched healthy controls and people with other psychiatric illnesses.[4] In this respect, iatrogenic metabolic effects of psychotropic drugs can be partly responsible, but these are not the only reason as cardiovascular risk factors such as raised body mass index and impaired glucose tolerance can occur even in the absence of pharmacotherapy.[5]

General medical comorbidities have a significant negative impact on illness with a more complicated course, increased cost of treatment and greater workplace disability. Mood disorder patients with three or more co-occurring medical conditions often have more severe mood episodes, increased suicidal behavior, poorer functioning, higher rates of co-occurring neuropsychiatric disorders and polypharmacy compared to people with no history of medical illnesses.[6] In addition, obesity, a chronic low-grade inflammatory condition, is associated with cognitive dysfunction in MDD and BD, with deficits in several domains including attention and psychomotor skills.[7] On the contrary, type 2 diabetes mellitus (T2DM) is associated with higher frequency of rapid cycling, chronic course, profound psychosocial impairment and decreased overall functionality in mood disorders.[8]

Currently, several aspects of the pathophysiology of mood disorders remain poorly understood, and possible reasons for the high prevalence of general medical comorbidities are largely unknown. Nonetheless, several studies have shown increased proinflammatory cytokine levels in the serum and cerebrospinal fluid in these patients.[9] Furthermore, there is postmortem pathological evidence of inflammation in the brains of patients with severe mood disorders. These observed alterations in inflammatory markers suggest immune dysfunction may be an important mechanistic link between affective illnesses and metabolic/inflammatory comorbidities. Interestingly, Bond et al. (2016) observed that raised body mass index predicted an inflammatory state in BD patients and also indicated depressive relapse in these subjects. Additionally, this association was a stronger predictor of inflammation than recent mood episodes, which also cause an increase in inflammatory markers.[10] Furthermore, factors of metabolic syndrome were accompanied by higher plasma levels of C-reactive protein (CRP) and transforming growth factor-beta (TGF-β) after starting pharmacotherapy in BD type II, signifying an independent association between mood disorders and inflammation.[11] As such, according to this evidence abnormalities of the immune system may be a key link between medical illnesses and mood disorders, whereby immune dysfunction may be increasing the morbidity and mortality in these conditions. Figure 3.1 schematically depicts this relationship between inflammation, general medical comorbidities and affective episodes.

It is worth mentioning that immune-inflammatory mediators influence pathways involved in mood, motivation, psychomotor activity and cognition. In humans, tryptophan is an essential amino acid that is a required substrate for serotonin biosynthesis. However, about 95% of the tryptophan is metabolized via the kynurenine pathway and the rate limiting step of this reaction is the enzyme, indoleamine 2, 3-dioxygenase (IDO). Proinflammatory cytokines like interleukin-1 beta (IL-1β), IL-6 and tumor necrosis factor-alpha (TNF-α) transcriptionally induce IDO in a variety of cells, including brain elements like neurons and microglia, thereby reducing the availability of tryptophan for serotonin synthesis. Because of this direct alteration of monoamine levels by the cytokines, inflammatory activation has been hypothesized as a possible contributor in mood disorders.[12]

In addition to medical comorbid conditions mentioned thus far, it is important to note that major mood disorders are often coupled with several neurological diseases, chief among which are migraine, idiopathic neuropathic pain, vertigo, dizziness and restless legs syndrome. There is emerging evidence implicating immune-inflammatory imbalance in the pathogenesis and progression of these diseases. For example, mood disorders and migraine may both be neuroprogressive conditions and accumulating data indicate that inflammatory activation mediated by proinflammatory cytokines may be the underlying neurobiological substrate of this association.[13] In view of the abovementioned observations, medical and neurological comorbid conditions linked to mood disorders may all be mediated by a persistent proinflammatory state in the body, and in the sections which follow this alleged connection is explored from different perspectives.

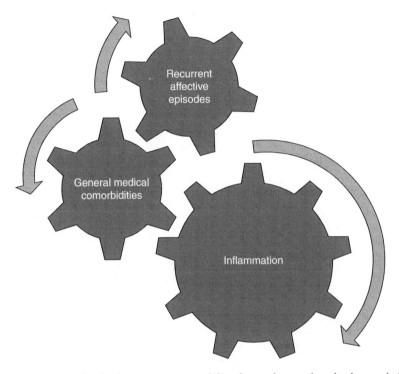

Figure 3.1 Role of inflammation in mood disorders and general medical comorbidities

In mood disorders there is a persistent low-grade inflammatory state that drives the pernicious process of disease advancement and likely results in chief medical abnormalities such as the metabolic syndrome, glucose intolerance and dyslipidemia. The key mediators are proinflammatory cytokines which are raised, and play an etiologic role in all of these conditions.

The Relation Between Mood Disorders and Inflammatory Comorbidities

Autoimmunity

Both MDD and BD are persuasively related to autoimmune diseases, including Guillain-Barré syndrome, autoimmune hepatitis, multiple sclerosis, rheumatoid arthritis, systemic lupus erythematosus, psoriasis and autoimmune thyroiditis.[14] Of these disorders, thyroid disease has a robust connection, particularly to BD. Although lithium treatment was suspected to have created this bias given the potential lowering effects of lithium on thyroid hormones, several studies have shown that BD may also be associated with thyroid disease independent of lithium use.[15] Thyroid autoimmunity may contribute to a rapid cycling course and compromise treatment response in bipolar patients. Additionally, various other pathogenic changes related to autoimmunity have been reported in mood disorders, including tendency towards

T helper cells 1, low T regulatory cells, senescence-related cell types and higher titers of autoantibodies.[16]

Hypersensitivity

Allergy is defined as increased sensitivity to innocuous antigens and may contribute to augmented risk of developing mood disorders, worsening of disease course and vice versa. For example, increased reactivity during the high pollen season exacerbates depressive symptoms in BD, while adolescents with asthma have a 2.2 times greater risk of developing BD and MDD in adult life than healthy controls[17]. Furthermore, co-occurrence of allergy enhances the risk of metabolic syndrome in patients with severe mental illnesses, including major mood disorders.

Chronic, Low-Grade Inflammation and the Metabolic Syndrome

Inflammation can be thought of as a process of tissue repair and protection which is initially produced by the innate immune system. Metabolic syndrome (MetS) is characterized by a cluster of risk factors for cardiovascular disease such as hypertension, hyperglycemia, dyslipidemia and obesity. To better comprehend the components of MetS, refer to Table 3.1 for the American Heart Association's criteria for MetS.

A persistent, low-grade inflammatory state is common in several medical disorders including MetS and a higher incidence of this condition is well documented in mood disorders.[18] As shown by Sicras et al. (2008), 24.7% of individuals with BD have some form of metabolic disease, while the percentage for the general population is 14.4%.[19] Additionally, both MDD and BD are more prevalent among individuals with obesity than without. Patients with BD have insulin resistance and higher blood glucose compared to healthy controls, which rises progressively with age. Furthermore, the risk of developing T2DM is three times higher in BD than in healthy controls; patients with unipolar depression are prone to the same abnormalities, albeit to a somewhat lesser extent.

Table 3.1 American Heart Association criteria for the metabolic syndrome (central obesity + any 2)

Parameter	Criterion
Waist circumference (cm)	>102 (M), >88 (F)
Blood pressure (mm Hg)	>130/85 (or undergoing treatment for HTN)
HDL (mmol/L)	<1.03 (M), <1.29 (F)
Triglyceride (mmol/L)	≥1.71
Glucose fasting (mmol/L)	≥5.5 (or undergoing treatment for DM)

DM – diabetes mellitus; HDL – high density lipoprotein; HTN – hypertension

Immune-Inflammatory Imbalance and General Medical Comorbidities

Reasons for the chronic activation of the immune system in mood disorders and its overall impact on general health may involve several aspects, both recognized and obscure. In this regard, inflammation provoked by MetS may act in concert with other factors and worsen the course of mood disorders. In obesity, hypertrophied adipocytes produce more leptin and less adiponectin and have infiltration of macrophages leading to systemic inflammation.[20] High density lipoproteins (HDL) act as anti-inflammatory agents by decreasing the secretion of TNF-α and IL-1β from activated monocytes, but HDL are low in dyslipidemia. Also, proinflammatory cytokines and high levels of free fatty acids promote insulin resistance. On the other hand, the existence of an inflammatory state in mood disorders may aggravate the risk for MetS. So far, it is not fully understood which exact pathways are incriminated, even though several biologically conceivable means have been identified. In reality, mood disorders may exacerbate immune dysfunction through several ways; next, the mechanisms of most significance are discussed. Table 3.2 provides a summary of factors that increase or decrease inflammation in affective illnesses and is helpful in understanding this association.

Table 3.2 Factors associated with increased or decreased inflammation in mood disorders

↑ *inflammation*	↓ *inflammation*
Genetic predisposition	Psychotropic medications – antidepressants, atypical antipsychotics, mood stabilizers
Psychological stress	Inflammation modulating agents – NSAIDs, ASA, celecoxib, omega-3 fatty acids, pioglitazone
Childhood maltreatment	Psychotherapy
Smoking/alcoholism/substance abuse	Healthy lifestyle
Obesity	Controlling factors associated with MetS
Sedentary lifestyle	Regular physical activity
Diet high in refined sugars, low in polyunsaturated fatty acids	Balanced diet/ following Mediterranean diet
Illness characteristics – repeated severe episodes, rapid cycling, persistent sub-threshold symptoms, psychosis	Electroconvulsive therapy
Intestinal dysbiosis, "leaky gut"	Probiotics, controlling factors associated with "leaky gut"

ASA – acetylsalicylic acid; MetS – metabolic syndrome; NSAIDs – non-steroidal anti-inflammatory drugs

Genetic Variations

Few studies have examined genetic variations in inflammation-related comorbidities and mood disorders, but initial results suggest these patients might carry genotypes predisposing to inflammation. For instance, compared to healthy individuals, BD patients have more genetic alterations in genes strictly related to pathways of IL-6, IL-8 and interferon-alpha (INF-α).[21] From 13 genes related to BD, *CASP1* and *STAT* were emphasized; the former is responsible for the production of IL-1β, while the latter encodes for a transcriptional factor that takes part in inflammatory responses. Genetic disparities in receptors of innate immunity have also been described in BD. For example, compared to controls, homozygous *TLR-4 rs1927914 A* and *TLR-4 rs11536891 T* alleles are common in BD, particularly in early onset cases and such disparity may be connected to decrease in effectiveness in protection against pathogens.[22] Moreover, there is low prevalence of *NOD2 rs2066482* polymorphism in BD, which may explain an association between Crohn's Disease and BD, and an earlier onset of inflammatory bowel disease in patients with BD compared with those without a lifetime history of a mood disorder.[23] Intriguingly, the *Val66Met* polymorphism in the brain-derived neurotrophic factor (BDNF) gene linked to suicidal ideation and higher stress responsiveness, is also correlated with raised body mass index in individuals without mood disorders.[24] This alludes to the fact that variations in key genes implicated in mood disorders give rise to well-recognized endophenotypes associated with affective illnesses.

Psychological Stress

Dysregulation of the hypothalamic–pituitary–adrenal (HPA) axis is well known in affective disorders. Several studies have shown that compared to controls, peripheral circulating levels of cortisol in MDD and BD subjects are abnormal during periods of euthymia, depression and mania. Glucocorticoid hormone values are higher in patients with rapid cycling, suicidal behavior and in those with multi-episodic course illnesses.[25] Persistent HPA activation leads to abnormal glucocorticoid signaling and blunted cortisol response. Glucocorticoid receptor (GR) activation has anti-inflammatory effects, but chronic stress can result in GR insensitivity preventing the negative feedback loop of the immune response. Additionally, inflammatory cytokines IL-1, IL-6, TNF-α and IFN-α lead to chronic hypercortisolemia by upsetting the negative feedback loop, which decreases HPA activity when an increased blood level of cortisol is detected. Hypercortisolemia has been shown to have several endocrine and metabolic effects including weight gain, insulin resistance and hypothyroidism, with adverse sequelae for people with a mood disorder.[26]

Childhood maltreatment and early childhood adversity are considered significant risk factors for elevated inflammatory cytokines and mood disorders. Within adult mood disorder patients, more than half testify to experiences of severe abuse during their childhood. These subjects appear to be more susceptible to bad prognostic features such as early onset, high frequency of episodes, psychotic symptoms and suicide attempts.[27] The immune system and the brain are not yet fully developed and have the highest plasticity during early life and thus can be severely affected by psychological stress. In this regard, defects in neuroplasticity resulting from epigenetic modifications, could be responsible for sustained inflammatory activation and consequent central and peripheral pathological responses.[28]

In individuals with or without mood disorders, history of abuse in childhood is coupled to increased inflammatory reactivity after psychological stress, compared to those who had not undergone such experiences. In addition, childhood trauma causes impairment in GR signaling and HPA axis hyperactivity, which reduces the ability of cortisol to decrease inflammation.[29] Furthermore, childhood maltreatment is linked to factors that increase inflammation such as gut microbiota imbalance, sleep disturbance, alcohol and substance abuse, autoimmune diseases and metabolic abnormalities.[30]

Substance Use

Comorbid substance use disorders are highly prevalent in mood disorders and are associated with an adverse impact on illness course. Underscoring this connection, in a large scale observational study approximately 58% of BD type I patients had alcohol use disorders and 37.5% had other drug use disorders.[31] Rates of smoking are also elevated in mood disorder patients which further provokes inflammation and causes oxidative and nitrosative stress. The induced increase in IgE antibodies and the cytokines TNF-α, IL-1, IL-6 and IL-8 by nicotine promotes conditions for both immune-suppression and autoimmune disorders.[32]

As already stated, mood disorders are highly associated with alcohol misuse and this has been implicated in reduced production of anti-inflammatory cytokines, such as IL-10 and increased synthesis of proinflammatory cytokines like TNF-α and IL-6 by cells mediating innate immunity. Furthermore, alcohol causes activation of nuclear factor-kappa B, a transcription factor involved in the maintenance of inflammatory response. Alcohol abuse leads to higher central adiposity, which further contributes to the continuation of a chronic proinflammatory state. Moreover, alcohol intake has significant effects on mood symptoms, even in the context of moderate consumption. Ethanol has the property of disrupting the blood–brain barrier, allowing increased brain exposure to cellular and biochemical mediators of inflammation, potentially contributing to the pathophysiology of mood disorders and increasing the risk for the related complication of suicidal behavior.[33]

The Gut–Brain Axis

In view of the emerging evidence about the function of gut microbiota in neurobiology and metabolic health, it is very likely that commensal bacteria may be a factor for activation of inflammation in mood disorders. Penetration of bacteria across the gut epithelium may result in persistent low-grade inflammation, which contributes to the metabolic abnormalities observed in chronic mood disorders. With regards to this alleged association, "leaky gut" was observed in MDD with increased concentrations of IgM and IgA as a defense induced by the endotoxin, lipopolysaccharide (LPS); however, this has yet to be replicated in a BD sample.[34] Interestingly, healthy humans have enhanced anxiety and depression, elevated plasma norepinephrine, salivary cortisol and proinflammatory cytokines after administration of LPS. To further advance this argument, dysfunction in gut microbiota may be associated with inflammation and metabolic syndrome in a bidirectional manner. According to DiBaise et al. (2008), intestinal microbiota is the possible mediating factor between inflammation and MetS induced by a high fat diet.[35] For instance, *Escherichia coli* may infiltrate the intestinal barrier and lead to low-grade systemic inflammation. Therefore, disturbance in the bacterial environment in the gastrointestinal tract is probably another relevant factor contributing to worse course of mood disorders and general medical comorbidities through inflammation.

Affective Episodes as Allostatic States

Recently, it has been assumed by some authors that mood episodes may act as a cause of toxicity and consequent inflammation.[36] This notion is held up by replicated evidence indicating a strong inflammatory state during mood episodes, especially during mania compared to depressive states and euthymia. Several original studies and some meta-analysis support the association between mania and a strong proinflammatory state, especially in unmedicated patients.[37] Euthymia and long-term treatment with the classical mood stabilizer, lithium, is associated with at least partial reversal of these abnormalities. While in the initial stages, euthymic periods are allegedly associated with reversion of immune-inflammatory changes; in multi-episodic affective illnesses there is an accumulation of these so-called "allostatic states", presenting a permanent challenge for the immune system. Continual immunological activation can exhaust the ability to adapt to changing physiological needs and return to homeostatic balance. The result is, besides enduring inflammation, impaired functioning of the adaptive immune system including increased vulnerability to infections and weaker responsiveness to anti-infective agents. To further extend this argument, one research group found preliminary evidence of accelerated aging of the immune system in mood disorder subjects, which was more noticeable in individuals with a history of multi-episode illness.[38] The allostatic load model of mood disorders and its relationship to general medical comorbidities is further elucidated with the help of Figure 3.2.

Role of Adipose Tissue

Of late, adipose tissue has been receiving attention in the field of mood disorder research and inflammation. Adipokines, cytokines secreted by adipose tissue,

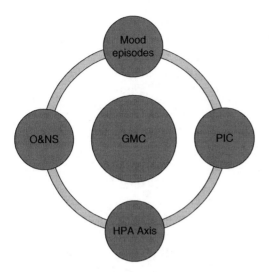

Figure 3.2 The relationship between mood episodes and general medical comorbidities

In mood disorders recurrent affective episodes act as allostatic states, causing derangement in hypothalamic–pituitary–adrenal (HPA) axis, raised proinflammatory cytokines and increased oxidative and nitrosative stress (O&NS). These factors purportedly play a causal role and lead to general medical comorbidities associated with major mood disorders.

have been evaluated in BD, especially adiponectin, resistin and leptin. Barbosa and collaborators (2012) reported that patients with BD had increased plasma levels of adiponectin and leptin compared to healthy volunteers.[39] Moreover, in the BD population adiponectin levels were correlated with fasting glucose, serum insulin, HDL and very low density lipoprotein (VLDL) cholesterol and triglycerides. After adjusting for age, gender and body mass index, individuals with BD and low adiponectin levels (i.e. < 7.5 μg/ml) had a significantly higher number of mood episodes, greater severity of depressive symptoms and lower levels of functioning. The authors of this study concluded that adiponectin levels, either directly or as an intermediary for metabolic dysfunction, are independently associated with an adverse illness course in BD.[40]

Therapeutic Considerations

Medication-Induced Metabolic Dysfunction

In the treatment of major mood disorders, atypical antipsychotics are used as first-line medications in BD and as adjuncts to standard antidepressants in MDD. These commonly used agents in the treatment of affective illnesses are shown to have an unfavorable effect on metabolic measures causing higher risk of obesity (2.5 times), glucose intolerance, dyslipidemia and weight gain.

Interestingly, some authors are skeptical about the harmful effects of new generation antipsychotics and advocate the view that these psychotropic drugs do not contribute to increased mortality in psychiatric patients.[41] In their opinion metabolic abnormalities are the consequence of systemic involvement, and this endorses the modern view that mood disorders are essentially multi-organ ailments afflicting not just the brain but the body as a whole.

Even so, according to the available data metabolic effects of second and third generation antipsychotics may be classified as high (clozapine and olanzapine), medium (iloperidone, paliperidone, quetiapine and risperidone) or low risk (aripiprazole, brexpiprazole, cariprazine, asenapine, lurasidone and ziprasidone).[42] Classical mood stabilizers, lithium and valproate, are associated with weight increase as well, and in this regard obese patients have a higher risk of medication-induced weight gain. Valproate may cause this side effect through increased craving for fatty foods. With respect to modern antidepressants, particularly selective serotonin reuptake inhibitors (SSRIs), long-term treatment may result in weight gain but several other variables must be taken into account and the jury is still out on the matter.[43] Nevertheless, metabolic side effects are just one aspect that should be taken into consideration in the medication selection process. Affective ailments are life-threatening conditions with potential negative consequences in the entire sphere of biopsychosocial functioning. Therefore, in the risk-benefit analysis when balancing safety with efficacy, it could be justified to use a drug associated with metabolic side effects, for example using clozapine for treatment-resistant patients, or lithium for its high efficacy and suicide preventing characteristics.[44]

Treating Mood Disorders and Comorbidities Together

An appraisal of the extant literature supports the notion that the psychiatric management and treatment of general medical comorbidities should be undertaken simultaneously. This synchronized approach is helpful in improving the overall outcome by ameliorating the affective symptoms, which has a salutary effect on general medical comorbidities as well, and psychotropic drugs are instrumental in this regard. The application of this strategy also apparently decelerates the process of neuroprogression, since general medical comorbidities are known to be associated with a chronic, relentless course in mood disorders. Obesity is a harbinger of inflammation and signifies treatment resistance to psychopharmacological interventions. As an example, mood stabilizers such as lithium and valproate are found to be less effective in patients with the metabolic syndrome.[45] Refractoriness to lithium is reported in diabetic BD patients, and more importantly there is a trend towards multiple treatment resistance in this population. In line with this evidence, it can be surmised that reducing body mass index and controlling the manifestations of MetS could potentially improve the responsiveness to the usual psychotropic agents in major affective illnesses.[46]

Using Anti-Inflammatory Agents in the Treatment of Mood Disorders

As inflammation is being increasingly incriminated in the pathophysiology of affective illnesses, research efforts are now directed at determining the value of anti-inflammatory agents in the overall management of these conditions. In a recent meta-analysis, adjunctive anti-inflammatory agents were shown to have antidepressant effects in BD.[47] Eight randomized controlled trials (RCTs; n = 312) assessing adjunctive non-steroidal anti-inflammatory drugs (NSAIDs, n = 53), omega-3 polyunsaturated fatty acids (n = 140), N-acetylcysteine (n = 76) and pioglitazone (n = 44) in the treatment of BD were included in the quantitative analysis. The overall effect size of adjunctive anti-inflammatory agents on depressive symptom severity was -0.40 (95% confidence interval -0.14 to -0.65, $p = 0.002$), indicative of a moderate and statistically significant antidepressant effect. Noticeably, the majority of studies included in this meta-analysis had small sample sizes and short trial durations, a design that is inclined to overrate treatment effects. Nonetheless, this meta-analysis is significant as it provides an unequivocal proof of efficacy and determines that additional, more robust studies evaluating immune-modulating agents are worth pursuing in subjects throughout the spectrum of mood disorders.

Furthermore, identifying subgroups of patients with disease characteristics that are more likely to respond to add-on anti-inflammatory treatments may also be very important. In BD, certain studies suggest improved efficacy of lithium or atypical antipsychotic when augmented by NSAIDs, acetylsalicylic acid and celecoxib, with the potential for decreased depressive symptoms and lowered relapse and recurrence rates.[48] A recently published review further advances this argument and suggests the efficacy of anti-inflammatory modalities in MDD cases is only in sub-populations with evidence of raised biomarkers of inflammation and is therefore not generalizable to all patients with the ailment. Important insights are provided by currently published case reports, for instance BD patients afflicted with psoriasis showed improvement in mood symptoms when treated with infliximab, a monoclonal anti-TNF-α antibody.[49] In addition, the same agent improved affective symptoms in a Crohn's disease patient who had a psychotic episode.[50] From another perspective, a large cohort study showed the use of sulfonylureas and metformin in the treatment of type II diabetes was associated with a decreased risk of developing affective disorders.[51] The antidepressant effect of rosiglitazone was reported in murine models, and in humans with unipolar or bipolar depression. Likewise, pioglitazone was recently shown to have an antidepressant effect in MDD and BD with or without MetS and caused no serious adverse effects in this population. However, there is a caveat: it is necessary to be aware of the risks of combining medications, such as lithium with NSAIDs which together can potentiate nephrotoxicity and as such should be avoided.

The Role of Regular Physical Exercise

Patients with major mood disorders have reduced frequency and intensity of physical activity, although the antidepressant properties of exercise might be beneficial in their overall management, with additional salutary effects on metabolic parameters and cardio-respiratory status.[52] Weight loss is generally associated with increased levels of BDNF, lowered proinflammatory markers and decreased severity of depressive symptoms. Subjects with BD, MDD and schizophrenia that undertook a program of dietary alterations, exercise and healthy lifestyle changes had lower waist circumference and better mental health after the trial.[53] Another study in BD subjects with a similar intervention reported reductions in weight, total cholesterol, triglycerides and glucose, as well as improvement in depressive symptomatology.[54]

Restoring Gut Microbiota Imbalance

Although research on the gut–brain axis is in its early stages, it is already becoming apparent that the resident bacteria in the gastrointestinal tract have a role in the pathophysiology of mood disorders. In this regard, probiotics or ingested beneficial microbes have been shown to increase expression of BDNF, while having significant modulatory effects on glutamatergic neurotransmission.[55] These organisms also modify the immune response in affective disorders and result in more self-tolerance and less hypersensitivity by increasing the function of regulatory T lymphocytes and an enhancement of the immune reactivity. In experiments in mice, the production of short chain fatty acids by symbiotic bacteria has a role in reducing inflammation and decreasing insulin resistance, while at the same time protecting the integrity of the blood–brain barrier. Moreover, the administration of probiotics, namely bifidobacterium lactis, streptococcus thermophiles, lactobacillus bulgaricus, and lactococcus lactis improves brain connectivity and emotional processing in healthy women; two of these (lactobacillus and bifidobacterium) have been shown to reduce stress and anxiety in healthy humans.[56] Figure 3.3 provides an overview of the treatment strategy described here regarding the management of general medical comorbidities in mood disorders.

Conclusion

General medical comorbidities are not just an aggregate of diverse factors, but rather represent an intricate alteration of biological pathways which act in a deleterious manner to negatively influence the course of mood disorders. The association could be causal, with mood exacerbations leading to inflammation and consequently general medical comorbidities. The metabolic syndrome can also negatively impact the progression of mood disorders. However, these could be two faces of the same coin, with immune dysfunction leading to both affective illnesses and general medical comorbidities. Because of higher illness

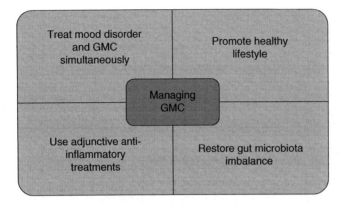

Figure 3.3 Treatment of general medical comorbidities in mood disorders

A wide-ranging therapeutic approach is advocated in managing mood disorder patients with general medical comorbidities. While there is mixed evidence with regards to using psychotropic medications with metabolic side effects, these are considered as very important in the overall management of mood disorders. In this regard, general medical comorbidities must be managed simultaneously along with the affective episodes. It is essential to promote a healthy lifestyle with balanced diet, regular physical activity and abstinence from alcohol and drugs of abuse. Using anti-inflammatory agents may be warranted in a subset of patients with raised inflammatory markers. With the emerging importance of the gut–brain axis in mental disorders, restoring gastrointestinal microbial imbalance may be significant in the general treatment.

severity in mood disorder patients with general medical comorbidities, a physically active lifestyle with avoidance of substance abuse is highly desirable, while to avoid iatrogenic effects using medications with less risk of derangement in metabolic parameters is recommended. Furthermore, anti-inflammatory medications may be of benefit; however, more research is required to confirm their efficacy in affective illnesses. Finally, managing mood disorders and general medical comorbidities simultaneously is an important strategy to enhance treatment outcomes for both. As an ending note, it is worth stating that further research efforts are necessary to enhance the understanding of the underlying mechanisms, and clarify results of interventions directed towards decreasing the burden of general medical comorbidities.

Summary Points

- Mood disorders are systemic conditions and are frequently associated with physical ailments of a chronic nature.
- Chief among these are metabolic abnormalities, cardiovascular diseases, immune-based and endocrine disorders.
- The excess morbidity and mortality associated with mood disorders is a result of general medical comorbidities.
- Several lines of evidence point to disturbance in inflammatory homeostasis in affective illnesses and the associated general medical comorbidities.

- Emerging evidence points to the presence of a persistent inflammatory state in the advancement of both conditions.
- The "leaky gut" hypothesis of mood disorders posits that disturbed balance in the commensal intestinal bacteria aggravates the course of mood disorders and also contributes to general medical comorbidities.
- There is some proof that modern psychotropic agents improve mood disorder symptomatology by reducing the chronic low-grade inflammation.
- Current premise holds that both mood episodes and general medical comorbidities should be treated simultaneously.
- Further therapeutic measures must include promotion of a healthy lifestyle including balanced diet, regular physical exercise, avoidance of substance use and restoration of the gut microbiota imbalance.

References

1) Laursen TM, Wahlbeck K, Hällgren J, Westman J, Ösby U, Alinaghizadeh H, et al. Life expectancy and death by diseases of the circulatory system in patients with bipolar disorder or schizophrenia in the Nordic countries. PLoS One 2013;8:e67133.
2) Kessing LV, Vradi E, McIntyre RS, Andersen PK. Causes of decreased life expectancy over the life span in bipolar disorder. J Affect Disord 2015;180:142–147.
3) Crump C, Sundquist K, Winkledy MA, Sundquist J. Comorbidities and mortality in bipolar disorder: a Swedish national cohort study. JAMA Psychiatry 2013;70:931–939.
4) Parikh SV, LeBlanc SR, Ovanessian MM. Advancing bipolar disorder: key lessons from the systematic treatment enhancement program for bipolar disorder (step-BD). Can J Psychiatry 2010;55:136–143.
5) Mansur RB, Brietzke E, McIntyre RS. Is there a "metabolic mood syndrome"? A review of the relationship between obesity and mood disorders. Neurosci Biobehav Rev 2015;52:89–104.
6) Forty L, Ulanova A, Jones L, Jones I, Gordon-Smith K, Fraser C, et al. Comorbid medical illness in bipolar disorder. Br J Psychiatry 2014;205:465–472.
7) Mansur RB, Ahmed J, Cha DS, Woldeyohannes HO, Subramaniapillai M, Lovshin J, et al. Liraglutide promotes improvements in objective measures of cognitive dysfunction in individuals with mood disorders: a pilot, open-label study. J Affect Disord 2017;207:114–120.
8) Calkin CV, Ruzickova M, Uher R, Hajek T, Slaney CM, Granham JS, et al. Insulin resistance and outcome in bipolar disorder. Br J Psychiatry 2015;206:52–57.
9) McNamara RK, Lotrich FE. Elevated immune-inflammatory signaling in mood disorders: a new therapeutic target? Expert Rev Neurother 2012;12:1143–1161.
10) Bond DJ, Andreazza AC, Hughes J, Dhanoa T, Torres IJ, Kozicky M, et al. Association of peripheral inflammation with body mass index and depressive relapse in bipolar disorder. Psychoneuroendocrinology 2016;65:76–83.
11) Lee SY, Chen SL, Chang YH, Chen PS, Huang SY, Tzeng NS, et al. Inflammation's association with metabolic profiles before and after a twelve-week clinical trial in drug-naïve patients with bipolar II disorder. PLoS One 2013;8:e66847.

12) Bradley KA, Case JA, Khan O, Ricart T, Hanna A, Alonso CM, et al. The role of the kynurenine pathway in suicidality in adolescent major depressive disorder. Psychiatry Res 2015;227:206–212.

13) Patten SB, Williams JV, Lavorato DH, Wang JL, Jette N, Sajobi TT, et al. Patterns of association of chronic medical conditions and major depression. Epidemiol Psychiatr Sci 2016; 1–9:[Epub ahead of print].

14) Bakunina N, Pariante CM, Zunszain PA. Immune mechanisms linked to depression via oxidative stress and neuroprogression. Immunology 2015; 144:365–373.

15) Krishna VN, Thunga R, Unnikrishnan B, Kanchan T, Bukelo MJ, Mehta RK, et al. Association between bipolar affective disorder and thyroid dysfunction. Asian J Psychiatr 2013;6:42–45.

16) do Prado CH, Rizzo LB, Wieck A, Lopes RP, Teixeira AL, Grassi-Oliveira R, et al. Reduced regulatory T cells are associated with higher levels of Th1/Th17 cytokines activated MAPK in type I bipolar disorder. Psychoneuroendocrinology 2013;38:667–676.

17) Chen MH, Su TP, Chen YS, Hsu JW, Huang KL, Chang WH, et al. Higher risk of developing major depression and bipolar disorder in later life among adolescents with asthma: a nationwide prospective study. J Psychiatr Res 2014;49:25–30.

18) Bortolasci CC, Vargas HO, Vargas Nunes SO, de Melo LG, de Castro MR, Moreira EG, et al. Factors influencing insulin resistance in relation to atherogenicity in mood disorders, the metabolic syndrome and tobacco use disorder. J Affect Disord 2015;179:148–155.

19) Sicras A, Rejas J, Navarro R, Serrat J, Blanca M. Metabolic syndrome in bipolar disorder: a cross-sectional assessment of a Health Management Organization database. Bipolar Disord 2008;10:607–616.

20) Yamagata AS, Mansur RB, Rizzo LB, Rosenstock T, McIntyre RS, Brietzke E. Selfish brain and selfish immune system interplay: A theoretical framework for metabolic comorbidities of mood disorders. Neurosci Biobehav Rev 2017;72:43–49.

21) Drago A, Crisafulli C, Calabro M, Serretti A. Enrichment pathway analysis. The inflammatory genetic background in bipolar disorder. J Affect Disord 2015;179:88–94.

22) Oliveira J, Busson M, Etain B, Jamain S, Hamdani N, Boukouaci W, et al. Polymorphism of Toll-like receptor 4 gene in bipolar disorder. J Affect Disord 2014;152–154:395–402.

23) Walker JR, Ediger JP, Graff LA, Greenfeld JM, Clara I, Lix L, et al. The Manitoba IBD cohort study: a population-based study of the prevalence of lifetime and 12-month anxiety and mood disorders. Am J Gastroenterol 2008;103:1989–1997.

24) Shugart YY, Chen L, Day IN, Lewis SJ, Timpson NJ, Yuan W, et al. Two British women studies replicated the association between the Val66Met polymorphism in the brain-derived neurotrophic factor (BDNF) and BMI. Eur J Hum Genet 2009;17:1050–1055.

25) Kamali M, Saunders EF, Prossin AR, Brucksch CB, Harrington GJ, Langenecker SA, et al. Associations between suicide attempts and elevated bedtime salivary cortisol levels in bipolar disorder. J Affect Disord 2012;136:350–358.

26) Aydin A, Selvi Y, Besiroglu L, Boysan M, Atli A, Ozdemir O, et al. Mood and metabolic consequences of sleep deprivation as a potential endophenotype in bipolar disorder. J Affect Disord 2013;150:284–294.

27) Melhem NM, Keilp JG, Porta G, Oquendo MA, Burke A, Stanley B, et al. Blunted HPA axis activity in suicide attempters compared to those at high risk for suicidal behavior. Neuropsychopharmacology 2016;41:1447–1456.

28) Teicher MH, Samson JA. Childhood maltreatment and psychopathology: A case for ecophenotypic variants as clinically and neurobiologically distinct subtypes. Am J Psychiatry 2013;170:1114–1133.

29) Lukic I, Mitic M, Soldatovic I, Jovicic M, Maric N, Radulovic J, et al. Accumulation of cytoplasmic glucocorticoid receptor is related to elevation of FKBP5 in lymphocytes of depressed patients. J Mol Neurosci 2015;55:951–958.

30) Grosse L, Ambree O, Jorgens S, Jawahar MC, Singhal G, Stacey D, et al. Cytokine levels in major depression are related to childhood trauma but not to recent stressors. Psychoneuroendocrinology 2016;73:24–31.

31) Grant BF, Stinson FS, Hasin DS, Dawson DA, Chou SP, Ruan WJ, et al. Prevalence, correlates, and comorbidity of bipolar I disorder and axis I and II disorder: results from the National Epidemiologic Survey on Alcohol and Related Conditions. J Clin Psychiatry 2005;66:1205–1215.

32) Arnson Y, Shoenfeld Y, Amital H. Effects of tobacco smoke on immunity, inflammation and autoimmunity. J Autoimmun 2010;34:258–265.

33) Brière FN, Rohde P, Seeley JR, Klein D, Lewinsohn PM. Comorbidity between major depression and alcohol use disorders: a unique patient population. Compr Psychiatry 2014;55:526–533.

34) Slyepchenko A, Maes M, Jacka FN, Köhler CA, Barichello T, McIntyre RS, et al. Gut microbiota, bacterial translocation, and interaction with diet: pathophysiological links between major depressive disorder and non-communicable medical comorbidities. Psychother Psychosom 2017;86:31–46.

35) DiBaise JK, Zhang H, Crowell MD, Krajmalnik-Brown R, Decker GA, Rittmann BE. Gut microbiota and its possible relationship with obesity. Mayo Clin Proc 2008;83:460–469.

36) McEwen BS. Mood disorders and allostatic load. Biol Psychiatry 2003;54:200–207.

37) Modabbernia A, Taslimi S, Brietzke E, Ashrafi M. Cytokine alterations in bipolar disorder: a meta-analysis of 30 studies. Biol Psychiatry 2013;74:15–25.

38) Rizzo LB, Do Prado CH, Grassi-Oliveira R, Wieck A, Corream BL, Teixeira AL, et al. Immunosenescence is associated with human cytomegalovirus and shortened telomeres in type I bipolar disorder. Bipolar Disord 2013;15:832–838.

39) Barbosa IG, Rocha NP, de Miranda AS, Magalhães PV, Huguet RB, de Souza LP, et al. Increased levels of adipokines in bipolar disorder. J Psychiatr Res 2012;46:389–393.

40) Mansur RB, Rizzo LB, Santos CM, Asevedo E, Cunha GR, Noto MN, et al. Adipokines, metabolic dysfunction and illness course in bipolar disorder. J Psychiatr Res 2016;74:63–69.

41) Khan A, Faucett J, Morrison S, Brown WA. Comparative mortality risk in adult patients with schizophrenia, depression, bipolar disorder, anxiety disorders and attention deficit/hyperactivity disorder participating in psychopharmacology clinical trials. JAMA Psychiatry 2013;70:1091–1099.

42) Hasnain M, Vieweg WV, Hollett B. Weight gain and glucose dysregulation with second-generation antipsychotics and antidepressants: a review for primary care physicians. Postgrad Med 2012;124:154–167.

43) Uguz F, Sahingoz M, Gungor B, Aksoy F, Askin R. Weight gain and associated factors in patients using newer antidepressant drugs. Gen Hosp Psychiatry 2015;37:46–48.

44) Malhi GS, Bassett D, Boyce P, Bryant R, Fitzgerald PB, Fritz K, et al. Royal Australian and New Zealand College of Psychiatrists clinical practice guidelines for mood disorders. Aust N Z J Psychiatry 2015;49:1087–1206.

45) Kemp DE, Gao K, Chan PK, Ganocy SJ, Findling RL, Calabrese JR. Medical comorbidity in bipolar disorder: relationship between illnesses of the endocrine/metabolic system and treatment outcome. Bipolar Disord 2010;12:404–413.

46) Kloiber S, Ising M, Reppermund S, Horstmann S, Dose T, Majer M, et al. Overweight and obesity affect treatment response in major depression. Biol Psychiatry 2007;62:321–326.

47) Rosenblat D, Kakar R, Berk M, Kessing RV, Vinberg M, Baune BT, et al. Anti-inflammatory agents in the treatment of bipolar depression: a systematic review and meta-analysis. Bipolar Disord 2016;18:89–101.

48) Nery FG, Monkul ES, Hatch JP, Fonseca M, Zunta-Soares GB, Frey BN, et al. Celecoxib as an adjunct in the treatment of depressive or mixed episodes of bipolar disorder: a double-blind, randomized, placebo-controlled study. Hum Psychopharmacol 2008;23:87–94.

49) Bassukas ID, Hyphantis T, Gamvroulia C, Gaitanis G, Mavreas V. Infliximab for patients with plaque psoriasis and severe psychiatric comorbidity. J Eur Acad Dermatol Venereol 2008;22:257–258.

50) Reimer J, Fink T, Blaker M, Schafer I, Otte C. Successful treatment of psychosis with infliximab in a patient with Crohn's disease. Schizophr Res 2009;109:194–195.

51) Wahlqvist ML, Lee MS, Chuang SY, Hsu CC, Tsai HN, Yu SH, et al. Increased risk of affective disorders in type 2 diabetes is minimized by sulfonylurea and met-formin combination: a population-based cohort study. BMC Med 2012;10:150.

52) Abdelhafiz AH, Sinclair AJ. Diabetes, Nutrition and Exercise. Clin Geriatr Med 2015;31:439–451.

53) Van Citters AD, Pratt SI, Jue K, Williams G, Miller PT, Xie H, et al. A pilot evaluation of the In SHAPE individualized health promotion intervention for adults with mental illness. Community Ment Health J 2010;46:540–552.

54) Sylvia LG, Sakedo S, Bernstein EE, Baek JH, Nierenberg AA, Deckersbash T. Nutrition, exercise, and wellness treatment in bipolar disorder: proof of concept for a consolidated intervention. Int J Bipolar Disord 2013;1:24.

55) Savignac HM, Corona G, Mills H, Chen L, Spencer JP, Tzortzis G, et al. Prebiotic feeding elevates central brain derived neurotrophic factor, N-methyl-d-aspartate subunits and d-serine. Neurochem Int 2013;63:756–764.

56) Messaoudi M, Lalonde R, Violle N, Javelot H, Desor D, Nejdi A, et al. Assessment of psychotropic-like properties of a probiotic formulation (Lactobacillus helveticus R0052 and Bifidobacteriumlongum R0175) in rats and human subjects. Br J Nutr 2011;105:755–764.

4   The Role of Epigenetics

Introduction

Major mood disorders like major depressive disorder (MDD) and bipolar disorder (BD) are common and multifaceted neuropsychiatric conditions, typified by a wide array of symptoms. These ailments cause extreme personal discomfort and result in profound impairment of functioning in all domains of life. In the diagnosis of mood disorders, the presenting symptoms should not be due to bereavement, a general medical condition or substance abuse. These must be present for a continuous period of at least two weeks in the case of a major depressive episode, whereas in mania there is no time limit if the patient requires hospitalization.[1] To explain the pathophysiology of mood disorders the classical monoaminergic hypothesis was put forward; however, recent research expounded two major assumptions based on dysfunction in the immune-inflammatory system (cytokine hypothesis) and neuronal plasticity in the brain (neurotrophic hypothesis).[2]

The cytokine hypothesis posits that, acting through inflammatory mechanisms severe and persistent environmental stressors, as well as organic inflammatory conditions, precipitate affective episodes.[3] Indeed, systemic infections, cancer or autoimmune diseases, in addition to stressful life events, are distinguished by the stimulation of the peripheral immune system. This is a prerequisite for the defensive reaction of the body against an ongoing challenge. However, when the activation of the immune system is protracted because of the persistence of the stressor, cytokines and other immune modulators are produced in an increasing amount and gain access to the brain where these disrupt the functioning of the organ and result in neuropsychiatric symptoms.[4]

The neurotrophic premise has gained precedence based on firm proof indicating that affective disorders may be linked to structural abnormalities in brain regions involved in emotional regulation. Furthermore, there is mounting evidence pointing to dysregulation in the communication between brain cellular elements, including neurons and glia. These changes may be reversible initially but become permanent with disease progression, such that effective therapeutic modalities should be instituted early to rectify the deficits in people with a mood disorder.[5] One reason for the neurotrophic hypothesis gaining ascendance is the fact that all effective treatments, whether psychopharmacological or behavioral, consistently increase the levels of the chief neurotrophic factor, i.e., brain-derived neurotrophic factor (BDNF).

The purpose of this chapter is to highlight the alterations in inflammation and neuronal plasticity that may be pertinent to the pathophysiology of mood disorders. However, it is worth remembering that the etiology of affective illnesses has been associated, at least in a subset of patients, with the experiencing of stressful events early in life. In this regard, it is very likely that inflammatory abnormalities and dysfunctional neuronal plasticity may underlie the persistent deleterious effects of early stressful life experiences, predisposing susceptible individuals to recurrent and severe affective disturbances.[6]

The Relationship Between Mood Disorders and Inflammation

Inflammatory Markers and Mood Episodes

There is an increasing amount of data indicating that mood episodes are linked to the triggering of the innate immune system.[7] This postulation has been reinforced over the last 20 years by a burgeoning body of evidence demonstrating that alterations occur in the functional activity of the immune system in mood disorder patients. To date, several studies have investigated blood and/or cerebrospinal fluid concentrations of one or more proinflammatory cytokines (e.g., interleukin-1 beta [IL-1β], IL-6, interferon gamma [IFN-γ]) or C-reactive protein (CRP); the latter is an acute phase protein which is raised in patients with major depressive, manic or mixed episodes.[8]

The bulk of these studies, whose principal findings have been recapitulated in several meta-analyses, report increased levels of IL-1β, IL-6, tumor necrosis factor-alpha (TNF-α) and CRP in the peripheral circulation of depressed and bipolar patients.[9] For instance, Hestad et al. (2003) showed that subjects with depressive disorders had markedly elevated TNF-α plasma levels compared with healthy controls.[10] Furthermore, akin to TNF-α higher plasma levels of IL-6, another proinflammatory cytokine, were demonstrated in comparable clinical samples. These findings were further consolidated by changes of cytokine mRNA levels during the investigation of peripheral blood cells. Actually, Tsao and colleagues found higher mRNA levels of TNF-α, IL-1β, IL-6 and interferon-alpha (INF-α) in the peripheral blood mononuclear cells (PBMCs) of patients with MDD.[11] In this regard, another group showed an increased expression of cytokine mRNA levels in the leukocytes of drug-free depressed patients as compared to controls.[12] Interestingly, identical cytokine abnormalities have been correlated with a number of clinical characteristics which portend worse prognosis and poor outcome. Of note, higher blood cytokines levels are linked to greater depression severity scores, as well as with inadequate antidepressant response to first-line agents. In this vein, increased CRP blood levels in MDD patients may serve as a biological signature of poor outcome to standard psychopharmacological strategies, a complicated course and poor outcome.[13]

Inflammatory Abnormalities in Adolescent Depression

Remarkably, initial findings have suggested a role for cytokines in child and adolescent depression which often has "melancholic" traits and carries an own burden of disadvantages, persisting or re-emerging in adulthood in major depressive and bipolar spectrum disorders.[14] Analogous to adult depression, an imbalance of the immune system epitomized by a disparity between proinflammatory and anti-inflammatory cytokines has been detected in adolescent depression. In this respect, increased levels of proinflammatory modulators, including IFN-γ, IL-6 and CRP have been found in depressed adolescents as compared to controls. Furthermore, such abnormalities have been discovered in youth with a history of childhood psychological or physical trauma.[15] In this group, the onset of depressive syndrome is characterized by a further increase of the proinflammatory markers and these remain elevated even after the improvement of the affective episode.[16]

Anomalies in the immune-inflammatory system occurring in unipolar depression and BD are also found in postmortem samples of brains of depressed suicide victims. Shelton and colleagues reported, for example, increased inflammatory pattern in the brains of depressed patients who committed suicide.[17] Likewise, recent studies in mood disorder subjects have identified abnormalities in protein and mRNA levels of toll-like receptors (TLRs), which play a role in neuronal functioning and result in increased production of cytokines and chemokines in response to inflammation or stress.[18]

Moreover, the incriminating role of inflammation in the pathogenesis of mood disorders has been upheld by the administration of proinflammatory agents like the bacterial endotoxin, lipopolysaccharide (LPS), which induces the development of depressive symptoms in humans.[19] To further extend this argument, around 30–40% of hepatitis C patients treated with the proinflammatory cytokine peg-interferon-alpha (pegINF-α) develop clinically significant depression. Last but not the least, major depression and bipolar disorder patients show increased comorbidity with numerous immune-related diseases such as cancer, cardiovascular and neurodegenerative disorders, which are all clinical conditions signified by the existence of inflammatory changes.

The Biological Mechanisms Linking Mood Disorders and Inflammation

Cytokines and the Brain

There are several paths through which cytokines can access the brain, influence central neuronal functioning and cause behavioral changes typified by the "sickness behavior". The latter is a corresponding set of psychological and physiological alterations that arise during the course of an infection and have similarity to the depressive phenotype.[20] One route may implicate mononuclear phagocytic cells sited at the circumventricular organs and the choroid plexus, which sense and react to circulating "pathogen-associated molecular patterns" by producing proinflammatory cytokines. Subsequently, these inflammatory modulators cross the blood–brain barrier, induce changes in neuronal functioning and result in the activation of microglia. A further way by which cytokines can influence the brain is via binding with their specific transporters, which are located on the blood–brain barrier.[21] Additionally, microglia cells in the brain express cytokine receptors, thus causing amplification of the inflammatory signals. Once in the brain tissue cytokines can control the working of this organ in a variety of ways, including the modulation of neurotransmitter metabolism and induction of neurotoxic pathways. For instance, cytokines induce the enzyme indoleamine 2,3 dioxygenase (IDO) which catalyzes the conversion of serotonin precursor, tryptophan, into kynurenine rather than 5-HT.[22] Once re-directed in this way, increasing amounts of quinolinic acid are produced which leads to neurotoxicity through the activation of the glutamatergic system.[23] Proinflammatory cytokines have also been shown to decrease neurotrophic support and to reduce neurogenesis in key brain areas, including the hippocampus. This may ultimately play a part in the decline of neuronal plasticity, a process that exemplifies an essential mechanism of mood disorder-related dysfunction.[24] Moreover, cytokines can increase the levels of stress hormones, including corticotrophin releasing hormone (CRH), adrenocorticotrophic hormone (ACTH) and cortisol, which have been reported to be elevated in patients with both MDD and BD and may consequently partake in HPA axis dysfunction, a fundamental disturbance in these neuropsychiatric disorders.[25]

Microglia Dysfunction

An increasing body of research incriminates deregulation of microglia function as important in neurologic and psychiatric diseases, since this may lead to critical changes in neuronal activity and working.[26] One main path through which microglia can modify brain functions related to psychiatric diseases is neurogenesis. The impact of inflammation on adult hippocampal neurogenesis was originally discovered by two separate groups (Ekdhal et al., 2003, and Monje et al., 2003), demonstrating that systemic or intrahippocampal administration of LPS reduced the formation of newborn neurons in the adult hippocampus, an effect that could be prohibited by indomethacin, a NSAID which acted by suppressing the synthesis of proinflammatory prostaglandins.[27]

Contingent on the inflammatory setting, microglia can wield a positive or negative influence on the proliferation, survival and differentiation of newborn neurons. For instance, these small mononuclear immune cells can compromise the neurogenic cascade during chronic stress, through the release of proinflammatory cytokines such as IL-1β, IL-6, and TNF-α.[28] During normal physiological conditions, microglia have been shown to engulf and destroy the excess of newborn neurons undergoing apoptosis in the hippocampal neurogenic niche. Moreover, a similar role for these elements has been suggested in the synaptic integration of newly formed cells, in the light of microglial cells phagocyting synaptic components.[29] In this respect, Kreisel et al. demonstrated a connection between stress-induced changes in microglia and the development of depression-like behavior in experimental conditions. Indeed, they showed a role of dynamic variations in microglia activation status in the development of chronic unpredictable stress (CUS)-induced depressive-like behavior in rodents. In the experimentation, the researchers demonstrated the ability of minocycline and of transgenic interleukin-1 receptor antagonist to rescue the subsequent microglial apoptosis, as well as the CUS-induced depressive-like behavior and suppressed neurogenesis.[30]

Importantly, depending on the activation state microglia may have opposite effects on adult neurogenesis in mammals, and it is likely that pro-neurogenic and anti-neurogenic microglial cells may coexist with different responsiveness to external stimuli. For instance, regular exercise such as voluntary running may have a positive effect and a pro-neurogenic phenotype of microglia, whereas adverse environmental conditions and aging result in the opposite effect. Therefore, it can be surmised that the overall outcome on adult neurogenesis may be determined by the result of the interaction between external factors and microglial state, mediated via inflammatory mechanisms.[31]

The Role of Psychotropic Medications

In the pharmacological treatment of mood disorders, cytokine variations have key implications with regards to response or otherwise to these interventions. A number of studies have shown the ability of some antidepressants to reduce cytokine activation in depressed patients. In this regard one research group recently demonstrated that cytokine expression in the leukocytes from depressed patients was reduced following escitalopram treatment, with a significant correlation between these changes and treatment response.[32] Furthermore, patients with major depression who are nonresponders to antidepressant therapies have higher plasma concentrations of proinflammatory cytokines and CRP as compared to responders.[33] In line with these findings, the Genome-based Therapeutic Drugs for Depression project (GENDEP) showed that patients who do not respond to two different classes of antidepressants have higher baseline mRNA levels of IL-1β, macrophage migration inhibitory factor and IL-6. Similar results on the role of TNF-α in the antidepressant treatment response have also been reported by the same group.[34]

It can be stated that peripheral inflammation conceivably modifies behavioral response to monoaminergic drugs, since elevated levels of cytokines are recognized to modulate monoamine synthesis, reuptake and metabolism, for instance by interfering with the function of the serotonin transporter which is a prime target of antidepressant drugs.[35] Accordingly, cytokine-induced alterations in monoaminergic signaling may not only bring on depressive states, but may also plausibly antagonize the therapeutic effects of monoamine reuptake inhibitors, triggering first-line treatment resistance. Likewise, monoaminergic drugs may exert a pharmacodynamic effect on inflammatory gene expression or peripheral immune cells, but this causality is still to be fully verified and substantiated.[36,37]

Neuronal Plasticity

Brain-Derived Neurotrophic Factor

Neuronal plasticity alludes to an array of mechanisms fundamental for brain functioning and represents the ability of this organ to perceive, adapt and respond to a range of internal and external stimuli. It is surmised that such mechanisms may be flawed in major psychiatric disorders and this defect may ultimately increase disease vulnerability.[38]

A great deal of evidence is indicative of the fact that stress, a major environmental precipitator of affective disturbances, can lead to an impairment of neuronal plasticity. Among the biological systems playing a crucial part in the maintenance of neuronal plasticity, neurotrophic factors and in particular the neurotrophin, BDNF, has emerged as a key mediator for proper functioning of brain elements.[39] Accumulating evidence now shows that decline in neurotrophic support is associated with deterioration in the biopsychosocial domains of functioning in patients with chronic mental illnesses. BDNF in actuality is not only essential during brain development, but it also exercises a central role in neuronal remodeling, as well as synaptic functioning throughout life. Several studies have revealed that in both BD and MDD patients the expression of BDNF is decreased in brain areas, such as the hippocampus and the prefrontal cortex, which represent the main anatomical targets for stress-induced structural alterations.[40] Preclinical studies have established the inverse relationship between stressful experiences and BDNF, since chronic exposure to different stress paradigms leads to a reliable decrease in this neurotrophin's expression. The values of BDNF are also reduced in the hippocampus and prefrontal cortex of "serotonin transporter knockout rats", a genetic model of depression and anxiety, signifying that variations in neuronal plasticity may play a part in the genetic vulnerability to mood disorders.[41]

Brain-Derived Neurotrophic Factor and Mood Disorders

Alterations in BDNF levels in mood regulating areas of the brain may be a significant factor in the expression of affective disorders. For instance, it has been demonstrated that targeted deletion of the BDNF gene results in behavioral dysfunction reminiscent of anxiety and depression, implying that such variations may contribute to the disease phenotype.[42,43] Moreover, BDNF expression plays a crucial role in resilience to chronic stress by participating in the formation and strengthening of neural connections involved in coping with such challenges. Since the levels of trophic factors are decreased in mood disorders, this abnormality may be implicated in psychosocial functional deficits associated with the said conditions. In this regard, it can be construed that effective pharmacological interventions would be able to stabilize such deleterious changes.

Brain-Derived Neurotrophic Factor and Psychotropic Medications

Certainly, a crucial phase in the long-term adaptive alterations brought about by psychotropic medications seems to be their capability of modifying the expression of BDNF as well as other growth factors. The bulk of the studies centering on BDNF have validated that first-line psychopharmacological agents used in the treatment of mood disturbances can affect BDNF transcription, translation and trafficking to specific sub-cellular compartments. Furthermore, BDNF receptor activation and signaling is also influenced by these medications.[44] Importantly, the ability to modulate BDNF has also been demonstrated for the rapid acting antidepressant ketamine which is an emerging strategy to manage refractory affective disturbances, most notably severe unipolar and bipolar depression and associated suicidal tendencies.[45] In this regard, it must be remembered that ketamine is not a traditional monoamine antidepressant, but rather represents a new class of drugs with pharmacodynamic effects on the glutamatergic pathway. To further extend this argument, a number of experimental studies have shown that dysregulated BDNF expression or release may undermine the antidepressants' action, implying that neurotrophin modulation may represent a significant mechanism of antidepressant drugs. This probability is in line with clinical data which show that serum BDNF levels which are decreased in depressed subjects, can be normalized only in patients that are responsive to pharmacological interventions.[46]

Brain-Derived Neurotrophic Factor and Neurogenesis

Alterations in BDNF levels result in functional and structural changes which impact brain regions key to affective disorders' pathogenesis and progression. An important effect that occurs downstream from neurotrophic factors is neurogenesis, the process by which neurons are created from stem cells. Certainly, chronic treatment with medications such as antidepressants, mood stabilizers and atypical antipsychotics does increase neurogenesis in the adult brain, primarily in the subgranular zone of the hippocampal dentate gyrus.[47] This mechanism is contingent on the regulation by trophic factors, and apparently plays a pivotal role in the beneficial, disease modifying actions of psychotropic drugs in mood disorder subjects.

Childhood Abuse and Mood Disorders

Childhood Maltreatment

Childhood trauma, which can be in the shape of physical, sexual or emotional abuse, is widespread in all communities and regions, and reported cases represent just the tip of the iceberg. In this regard, a recent meta-analysis shed light on the psychiatric consequences of childhood maltreatment. It showed that emotional abuse and neglect was strongly associated with depression, whereas sexual trauma, physical abuse and domestic violence were significantly correlated with later life psychological problems.[48]

Childhood maltreatment can be construed as acts committed by parents or caregivers knowingly or inadvertently, with resulting imminent harm to the child's health. Considering validated reports, 60% of the childhood maltreatment can be categorized as neglect, 20% as physical abuse and 10% as sexual abuse.[49,50] The occurrence of emotional abuse and neglect is expectedly much higher than that of sexual and physical maltreatment, but is nonetheless more problematic to measure and quantify. Based on the Childhood Trauma Questionnaire, Table 4.1 clarifies the types of maltreatment that are frequently found and measured in research and clinical settings.

The Relationship Between Early Life Trauma and Mood Disorders

A plethora of studies have demonstrated that the onset of mood disorders, such as MDD, is predisposed by stressful life events that occur in childhood. In an interesting study conducted in a community sample of young adults (ages 18–25), it was found that future occurrence of MDD and suicidal ideation was

Table 4.1 Classification of childhood trauma (Childhood Trauma Questionnaire)

Trauma subtype	Definition
Emotional neglect	Failure of caretaker to meet child's basic emotional and psychological needs including love, belonging, nurturance and support.
Emotional abuse	Verbal assaults on a child's sense of worth or well-being or any humiliating or demeaning behavior directed toward a child by an adult or older person.
Physical neglect	Failure of caretaker to provide for a child's basic physical needs including food, shelter, clothing, safety and health care.
Physical abuse	Bodily assaults on a child by an adult or older person that posed a risk of or resulted in injury.
Sexual abuse	Sexual contact or conduct between a child younger than 18 years of age and an adult or older person.

dependent on the particular age and specific type of childhood maltreatment. In that study, the most sensitive age was 14 years in both males and females, whereas non-verbal emotional abuse in boys and peer emotional abuse in girls were significant predictors of later psychopathology.[51] It is, therefore, obvious that diverse forms of child abuse have long-term negative results for mental health. Among the varied types of maltreatment, sexual abuse is undoubtedly the most significant with regards to increased risk for psychiatric disorders and suicidal behavior.[52] On the basis of these arguments, there is indeed a great deal of interest in understanding the mechanisms whereby exposure to adversities early in life leads to increased susceptibility to affective disturbances.

The Link Between Childhood Trauma and Inflammation

Human Studies

While the relationship between early life stressful events and mood disorders may be explained by several biological processes, a growing number of studies point towards a role for inflammation or enhanced responsiveness to inflammatory processes.[53] The Dunedin Multidisciplinary Health and Development Study is a large scale prospective study investigating the relationship between childhood trauma and later life depression. Taking advantage of the Dunedin cohort subjects, Danese et al. were the pioneers in showing that raised CRP blood levels were significantly associated with maltreatment during childhood and this connection was specifically robust in individuals who developed later life depression.[54] A recently published systematic review is helpful in understanding the association between childhood maltreatment and later life adverse conditions like obesity, diabetes and mental disorders. It demonstrated the presence of a chronic inflammatory state in victims of childhood abuse evidenced as raised circulating levels of CRP, fibrinogen and proinflammatory cytokines.[55] Furthermore, it was shown that depressed patients with a history of childhood abuse displayed an exaggerated inflammatory reaction when re-exposed to an acute psychological stress in adulthood, as specified by a heightened IL-6 response. In the same study, depressed subjects had enhanced DNA binding of the key proinflammatory transcription factor, nuclear factor kappa-light-chain-enhancer of activated B cells (NF-κB) in PBMCs.[56]

Hypothetical Framework

Based on this evidence, it is reasonable to speculate that individuals who experience major stressors early in childhood are more vulnerable to immune dysregulation in adult life, irrespective of whether they subsequently develop adverse physical or mental health consequences. In this respect, some leading researchers in the field have offered a model that presumes stress occurring during a sensitive period in life, when the immune function is under a great deal of flux, gets rooted in the functioning of the cells controlling the inflammatory process.[57] Hence, inflammatory cells such as macrophages, microglia and dendritic cells become highly sensitized resulting in a chronic proinflammatory state. This may be secondary to the activation of proinflammatory transcription factors such as NF-κB and downregulation of anti-inflammatory transcription factors such as the glucocorticoid receptor (GR), thereby enhancing the levels of circulating cytokines.[58] Furthermore, transformed reaction of innate immune cells to stimuli induces irregularities in other leucocytes, particularly T cells and B cells, which coordinate the adaptive immune responses. How childhood trauma produces a "proinflammatory phenotype" is hitherto an unresolved query, but is likely the consequence of deregulation in the highly intricate networks within biological pathways influenced by such experiences. In this regard, the investigation of epigenetic processes holds significant potential, since these operate at the interface between an individual's genetic background and his or her environment.[59] Figure 4.1 is an illustrative portrayal of the understanding that early life stresses produce epigenetic

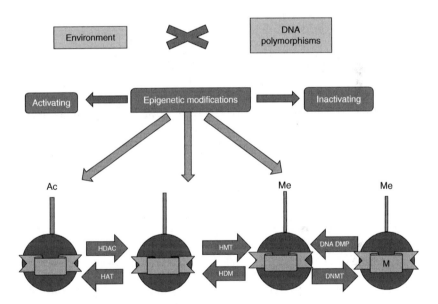

Figure 4.1 Epigenetic regulation of the mammalian genome

The pathogenesis of major mood disorders is explained through the interaction of environmental stressors acting on genetically transmitted vulnerabilities in susceptible individuals (gene x environment disorders). Epigenetic alterations can explain the way in which this interaction is expressed as specific phenotypes, such as major depressive disorder or bipolar disorder. Illustrated in Figure 4.1 is a simplified model of how reversible epigenetic modifications regulate transcriptional activity of genes. Acetylated histones (Ac) are associated with highly active genes, whereas methylation of histones (Me) at specific lysine residues (e.g., H3K9 or H3K27) is an inactivating signal. Methylation of cytosines at CpG dinucleotides in DNA (M) is also inactivating. Thus, epigenetic modifications can alter the expression of particular genes (e.g., BDNF) which are crucial in brain functioning and lead to specific psychiatric syndromes.

DNA DMP – DNA demethylation pathways; DNMT – DNA methyltransferase; HAT – histone acetyltransferase; HDAC – histone deacetylase; HDM – histone demethylase; HMT – histone methyltransferase

Circles represent histones, banners represent DNA.

alterations that result in the modulation of the functioning of crucial genes that play a key role in mood disorders.

Rodent Experiments

Experiments with rodents have demonstrated that early life stress induces an untimely stimulation of the immune system that can significantly sway the developmental trajectory of microglia, modifying the long-term activation pattern of these cells. As a result of such alterations, rats exposed to stress early in life are more susceptible to an upsurge in proinflammatory cytokine production following an LPS challenge in adulthood, signifying that the pro-inflammatory state continues in time and results in an elevated vulnerability and sensitivity to novel insults during adulthood.[60,61]

Childhood Trauma and Neuronal Plasticity

Early Life Maltreatment and Brain-Derived Neurotrophic Factor

Indeed, neuronal plasticity plays a key role in structural modifications in crucial brain areas, as a response to experiential learning and contributes to the ability to respond or adapt to environmental challenges. It is, therefore, reasonable to assume that changes in these processes may also underlie the long-lasting effects of adverse experiences occurring early in life.[62] In line with this probability, a persistent decrease of BDNF expression and function may characterize a collective endpoint for negative influences operating in early life. While such changes definitely occur, the anatomical specificity of these modifications is contingent on the type, timing and duration of the stressful event.[63]

Rodent Models

Experiments with rodents have shed light on the neuroplasticity process. For example, BDNF mRNA levels were decreased in the hippocampus of adult rats that were subjected to 24 h of maternal deprivation at postnatal day 9, while the application of more drawn out stressors during gestation or the early postnatal life (e.g., prenatal stress or repeated maternal deprivation) diminished the levels of the neurotrophin, mainly in the prefrontal cortex.[64] The time course study of BDNF alterations in rats subjected to prenatal stress (PNS) indicates that the decreased expression of BDNF seen in adult animals is not directly related to stress exposure, but is reliant on the maturational stage of the prefrontal cortex, becoming completely apparent after adolescence. Intriguingly, lurasidone treatment (a multi-receptor second generation antipsychotic) in adolescence prevented the neuroplastic dysfunction and had long-term beneficial effects on the developing brain.[65]

Brain-Derived Neurotrophic Factor Transcription and Translation

It must be appreciated that the expression of BDNF is under tight control to regulate its multifaceted actions in directing neuronal functioning. Transcription of BDNF is initiated from multiple promoters in reaction to disparate activation signals. Nevertheless, irrespective of which promoter is used, all BDNF transcripts are processed at two different polyadenylation sites, producing two pools of mRNAs that carry either a long or short 3' untranslated region (3' UTR).[66] The short 3' UTR BDNF mRNAs are confined to the soma or body of neurons, while the long 3' UTR mRNAs are predominantly localized in the dendrites.[67] Interestingly, it has been shown that exposure to PNS leads to a significant down regulation of the pool of BDNF transcripts. The long 3'UTR BDNF mRNA which is trafficked to the dendrites is particularly involved and its selective decrease after PNS may contribute to neuronal dysfunction with deficits in pruning and maturation of dendritic spines, as well as selective impairment of long-term potentiation in these locations.[68] Therefore, this phenomenon may contribute to impaired cell–cell communication and dysregulated synaptic function, eventually leading to cognitive and emotional deterioration evident after exposure to early life adversities.[69]

Brain-Derived Neurotrophic Factor Dysregulation and Reduced Neurogenesis

Remarkably, decreased neurogenesis was also discovered as a consequence of early life stress. For instance, PNS in rats brought about a lifespan decline in neurogenesis in the dentate gyrus and lead to an impairment of hippocampal-related spatial tasks.[70] In humans PNS can compromise learning with a focus on hippocampus-dependent operations, suggesting that the particular deficits arise from impaired formation of new neurons in the neurogenic niche of this organ.[71] Furthermore, in experimental paradigms the inhibition in neurogenesis has been shown to be associated with increased HPA axis activity and behavioral profiles suggestive of the depressive phenotype.[72]

Hypothalamic–Pituitary–Adrenal Axis Dysfunction

Rodent studies demonstrate that exposure to prolonged, rather than brief, bouts of maternal separation during the first two weeks of life results in a long-lasting suppression of adult neurogenesis and diminished plasticity in the hippocampus. More specifically, a decrease in cell proliferation and immature neuron production was observed in the dentate gyrus of adult rats subjected to stress that were maternally separated as pups.[73] Although the experimental animals showed normal basal levels of corticosterone (the main circulating glucocorticoid in rodents), the inhibition of cell production could be reversed by lowering corticosterone below the control value. Moreover, the usual stress-induced suppression of cell proliferation and neurogenesis, despite normal activation of the HPA axis, was not observed in maternally separated rats.[74] These observations suggested that stressors which acted in early life inhibited structural plasticity via hypersensitivity to glucocorticoids and diminished the ability of the hippocampus to respond to stress in adulthood. An interesting series of experiments demonstrated that rats exposed to a combination of valproate and lurasidone had greater increase in hippocampal BDNF levels than either drug alone and this effect was mediated in part by the regulation of histone deacetylases, signifying that some of the transcriptional changes were controlled by epigenetic mechanisms.[75]

The Epigenetic Link

Epigenetic Regulation of the Genome

By "epigenetics" is meant the persisting alterations in gene expression without changes of the DNA sequence, which are consequent upon numerous conceivably reversible processes comprising DNA methylation, histone modifications and aberrant expression of micro-ribonucleic acid (miRNA).[76] Included in the diverse array of epigenetic changes, DNA methylation is one of the best described mechanisms in relation to early life adversities.[77] No doubt, variations of DNA methylation at sensitive gene promoters may explain the continuation of the effects of early life trauma into adulthood which renders the afflicted subjects susceptible to ensuing insults and challenges.[78] In man, DNA methylation occurs almost entirely via covalent modification of DNA, in which methyl groups are coupled to cytosine residues of "CpG dinucleotides". DNA methylation has been demonstrated to be connected to alterations in gene expression, thereby operating as a potential mechanism for governing the transcriptional response to extracellular events. Figure 4.2 is an illustrative rendition of the link between early life stressful experiences, epigenetic alterations resulting in gene silencing or expression, and the expression of neuropsychiatric disorders.

Animal Studies

Many preclinical studies have underlined how contact with environmental stressors can result in persisting behavioral changes influencing survival capabilities through epigenetic modifications, mainly via changes in DNA methylation within certain designated brain regions. For instance, in rodents absence of maternal care leads to sustained deficits in the offspring, an anxious phenotype and elevated corticosterone levels in response to stress. These biobehavioral anomalies are linked to decreased hippocampal expression of GR which most likely represents the consequence of increased methylation at the GR gene promoter.[79,80] Furthermore, maternal separation in mice conceivably brings about hypomethylation in the vasopressin gene enhancer region, and this results in enhanced expression of hypothalamic vasopressin, accompanied by increased corticosterone secretion.[81]

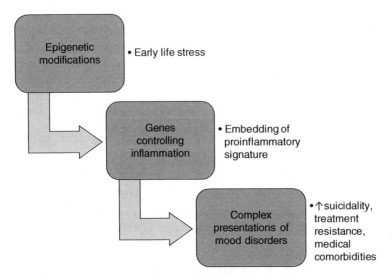

Figure 4.2 Early life trauma and its effect on adult presentations of mood disorders

Subjects who are exposed to traumatic events in childhood, in particular severe emotional, physical and sexual abuse are highly susceptible to developing affective disturbances which are complex and challenging to manage. The epigenetic modification of the genome is the link mediating the vulnerability between the genes and the environment. This area of research has the potential to uncover mechanisms underlying the multifaceted aspects of mood disorders and lead to new therapies which have actual curative value.

Human Studies

Intriguingly, similar changes have also been found to take place in humans. In this regard, studies in human postmortem brain showed early life traumatic experiences were related to increased methylation of the GR exon 1F promoter site in the hippocampus. Indeed, it must be understood that hippocampal GR activation regulates HPA activity and human GR expression is reduced in the hippocampus of suicide completers with a history of childhood abuse compared with controls.[82] In their study comparing brains of victims of suicide with a history of childhood abuse to suicide completers without such a background, Labonte et al. (2012) were able to further extend these findings. They demonstrated decreased levels of GR mRNA, as well as mRNA transcripts bearing the GR 1F splice variant and increased cytosine methylation of the promoter. Additionally, there was differential expression and methylation of GR exon 1(B), 1(C) and 1(H) in suicide completers with a history of childhood abuse.[83] These observations ostensibly validated the hypothesis that care giver abuse in childhood resulted in epigenetic deregulation of GR hippocampal expression, supporting the "translational" implications of exposure to early life stress in humans.

Epigenetic Modification of Neuroplasticity

Accumulating evidence indicates that in addition to the stress-response system, neuroplastic genes are also subject to epigenetic regulation, and this mechanism may be incriminated in the phenotypic expression of psychiatric illnesses.[84] In one study, rodent experiments revealed that the continued decrease in BDNF levels in the social defeat stress paradigm was secondary to epigenetic alterations in the promoter region of two of its transcripts in the hippocampus, resulting from repressive histone methylation of the latter.[85] In this vein, another group of investigators showed the expression of BDNF was significantly reduced in the prefrontal cortex of "serotonin transporter knockout rats" through an increased methylation in the promoter region of exons VI and reduced H3 acetylation at exon IV of the neurotrophin's gene.[86] While shedding light on the molecular mechanisms of depression under serotonin transporter dysfunction, these findings were in accordance with human postmortem studies as increased BDNF promoter methylation had been discovered in the brain of suicide subjects.[87] It could be further assumed that such modifications might also exemplify the result of early life adversities. Certainly, abuse during infancy in rodents resulted in a sustained increase of methylation in BDNF exon-4 and exon-9 that gave rise to reduced neurotrophin expression in the adult prefrontal cortex.[88] A recent study further strengthened these findings by examining changes in global levels of DNA methylation (5-mC) and hydroxymethylation (5-hmC), as well as specific changes in the BDNF gene within the adolescent amygdala and hippocampus of caregiver maltreated rats.[89] It showed that while young females exposed to abuse exhibited no significant alterations in global 5-mC or 5-hmC levels, investigation of BDNF gene methylation revealed that maltreated females had greater methylation of exon IV DNA in the amygdala and ventral hippocampus. Whereas, adolescent males exposed to maltreatment showed no significant alterations in BDNF DNA methylation, and abused males had significantly higher 5-mC levels in the dorsal hippocampus and lower 5-hmC levels in the amygdala. These results established that the effects of the early caregiving environment were evident in the adolescent brain at the level of the epigenome, with brain-region specific and sexually-dimorphic epigenetic consequences that could have relevance to adolescent mental health and behavior.

The Epigenetic Basis of Mood Disorders

Importantly, an ever increasing number of studies are shedding light on the effects of early life stress on DNA methylation at the genome-wide level in the brain as well as in peripheral tissues.[89] These efforts are helpful in ascertaining biosignatures that may be linked to the long-term pathologic consequences of early life traumatic experiences.[90] In this regard, epigenetic modifications in the peripheral tissues may compare to a certain degree with changes in the brain.[91] As an example, differential rearing conditions of rhesus macaques was related to distinctive methylation in early adulthood in both the brain and T cells, implying that the reaction to early life adversity was system-wide and genome-wide and continued to adulthood.[92] Moreover, the finding that such DNA methylation variations were not restricted to the brain but could be found in the peripheral systems indicated that these alterations were also of pertinence to additional health problems, such as the increased risk for cardiovascular and metabolic diseases found in mood disorders.[93] In this regard, it will be highly important to examine and identify traces of inflammatory-immune methylation as a result of early life stress. This will ultimately furnish essential information for the connecting role of epigenetic alterations and inflammatory processes in the causation of mental illnesses and also serve to elucidate the comorbidity of affective disorders with different medical conditions.[94] Figure 4.3 conceptualizes the emerging understanding of mood disorders and provides a schematic version of the current pathogenic model.

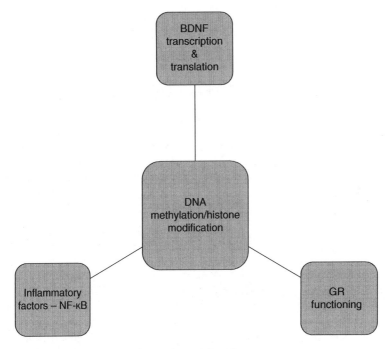

Figure 4.3 The epigenetic basis of mood disorders

The prevailing assumption on the pathogenesis of mood disorders states that these are gene x environment conditions. It is now suggested that situational adversities act in concert with inherited genetic polymorphisms causing lasting epigenetic changes and leading to the phenotypic expression of affective disorders. Among the key genes effected by early life adversity are the glucocorticoid receptor (GR), brain-derived neurotrophic factor (BDNF) and inflammatory transcription factors like the nuclear factor kappa-light-chain-enhancer of activated B cells (NF-κB). See text for further details.

Future Directions

The Significance of Epigenetic Regulation

As reviewed in this manuscript, there is convincing proof connecting early life stressful events, inflammation and neuroplastic abnormalities with affective disturbances, even though the fundamental biological mechanisms still need to be clarified. Emphasized here is the emerging role of epigenetics, and in particular of DNA methylation as one such underpinning mechanism. To recapitulate, among the most extensively studied paths of epigenetic regulation are DNA methylation, histone modifications and non-coding RNAs. However, because of its stability and ease of measurement, DNA methylation has been the most often studied. No doubt, early life stressful events can trigger epigenetic processes at global levels of the genome as well as at the promoter regions of key target genes, bringing about enduring and stable changes in gene expression which continue up to adulthood and may be responsible for an enhanced susceptibility towards developing psychiatric disorders. It must be understood that biological mechanisms that can integrate various hypotheses for the pathogenesis of mood disorders must fit certain paradigms, including:

1) ability to induce stable changes in physiology,
2) plasticity and responsiveness to both environment and genetic factors, and
3) capability to reconcile genetic and environmental contributions to disease.

Persistent epigenetic changes represent a conceivable contender for such an appreciation of the development of major mood disorders. In this respect, an improved knowledge may lead to the discovery as to how epigenetic changes impact on particular genes and contribute to the pathogenesis of major mental illnesses.

Inflammation as a Likely Epigenetic Mechanism

Increased inflammation is seen in many patients with mood disorders, and especially in those who do not respond to first-line psychopharmacological agents. Childhood adversity predisposes individuals to a stress-vulnerable phenotype marked by clustering of affective disturbances and inflammation. This is linked to sustained alterations in the behavioral, neuroendocrine and immune systems, three highly integrated allostatic neurobiological stress-responsive systems that detect and respond to environmental challenges. One potential mechanism by which increased risk for mood disorders occurs is epigenetic embedding of the inflammatory pathways. As such, future research should be able to explain whether increased inflammation truly reflects a single group of patients who had experienced childhood maltreatment, and manifested severe and treatment refractory forms of mood disorders. In this respect, inflammatory biomarkers may be useful in identifying and treating this sub-population of patients, as they are also likely to derive benefit from drugs that target inflammatory mechanisms.

Epigenetics and Neuroplasticity

BDNF has a central role in neuronal development and neuroplasticity, and its malfunctioning is implicated in a range of neurodegenerative and psychiatric disorders. The rapid pace of research in the epigenetic modifications and mechanisms controlling BDNF gene expression indicates that progress in BDNF epigenetics will have widespread applications in diagnosis, prognosis and biomarkers for psychiatric disorders. In this regard, it is worth remembering that DNA methylation exemplifies a stable epigenetic modification during early development, and at the same time signifies an important mechanism in experience-driven changes in the brain. It is proposed that activity-modified changes in DNA methylation may not affect transcription directly, but rather engender structural changes at the genomic locus that alter the transcriptional response to future stimuli, e.g., by changing the relative expression of alternative splice variants. Furthermore, with respect to the epigenetic regulation of BDNF, direct and indirect effects of DNA methylation are potential targets of therapy. To reduce nonspecific effects, targeted repair of epigenetic deregulation may be achieved through use of small interfering RNAs or by sequence-specific DNA-binding proteins linked to epigenetic modifying enzymes. Likewise, accumulating evidence suggests that epigenetic mechanisms are involved in the action of antidepressants, mood stabilizers and psychotherapy at the human BDNF gene promoter. DNA methyltransferase and histone deacetylase inhibitors, currently being tested in clinical trials for cancer treatment, could have applications in treating psychiatric disorders. Besides, epigenetic profiling of BDNF is applicable in both diagnosis and prediction of treatment response in psychiatric patients. Corresponding strategies include targeting the pathways involved in BDNF signaling, such as the TrkB receptor or the epigenetic regulation of BDNF via the methyl CpG (MeCP2) proteins.

Epigenetic Modification of HPA Axis Functioning

Finally, future studies should also provide novel understandings on the reversibility of the damage associated with childhood stressful experiences. The early life social environment can induce stable changes that influence neurodevelopment and mental health. The HPA axis is sensitive to changes in the early life environment that associate with DNA methylation of a neuron-specific exon 17 promoter of the GR (NR3C1). While stress responses and related outcomes vary markedly across individuals, elucidating the molecular underpinnings of this variability is of great relevance for developing individualized prevention strategies and treatments for stress-related disorders. An important modulator of stress responses is the FK506-binding protein 51 (FKBP5/FKBP51). FKBP5 acts as a co-chaperone that modulates not only GR activity in response to stressors but also a multitude of other cellular processes in both the brain and periphery. Notably, the FKBP5 gene is regulated via complex interactions among environmental stressors, FKBP5 genetic variants, and epigenetic modifications of glucocorticoid-responsive genomic sites. These interactions can result in FKBP5 disinhibition that has been shown to contribute to a number of aberrant phenotypes in both rodents and humans. Consequently, FKBP5 blockade may hold promise as treatment intervention for stress-related disorders, and recently developed selective FKBP5 blockers show encouraging results in *in-vitro* and *ex-vivo* rodent models. Although risk for stress-related disorders is conferred by multiple environmental and genetic factors, the findings related to FKBP5 illustrate how a deeper understanding of the molecular and systemic mechanisms underlying specific gene-environment interactions may provide insights into the pathogenesis of stress-related disorders. As a concluding note, future studies should elucidate whether pharmacological and non-pharmacological interventions could revert back the aberrations induced by childhood adversities on the functioning of systems involved in physiological responses. Such research should suggest strategies to minimize the risk for mood disorders, both in the individuals affected and in the next generations.

Conclusion

While it is widely recognized that mood disorders are gene x environment disorders, the exact genes responsible for this vulnerability have not been established even after decades of research. Nonetheless, significant insights have been developed and it is now known that these are polygenic disorders and specific genes bearing biosignatures of adverse early environmental influences contribute to the expression of psychiatric diseases. Epigenetic alterations exemplified by DNA methylation, histone modifications and non-coding RNAs serve as the mediating link in this respect. These changes can be identified at the candidate gene and genome-wide levels and lead to dysregulation of key systems involved in stress responsiveness. Emerging evidence points to the inflammatory-immune system, BDNF and HPA axis, which acting in concert bring about the neuropsychiatric and systemic manifestations of affective illnesses. Elucidation of the epigenetic mechanisms has the potential to lead to the development of new treatment strategies with far reaching benefits to the patients.

Summary Points

- Since almost half the adults with mood disorders recollect childhood experiences of maltreatment, it is important to investigate paths through which early stressful events cause psychopathological disturbances in later life.

- Childhood psychological, physical and sexual abuse is common in all societies and cultures and recent systematic reviews and meta-analyses show this has adverse consequences for both mental and bodily health.
- In susceptible individuals, environmental stressors acting on specific genes can result in potentially reversible alterations of the genome, referred to as "epigenetic" modifications.
- These lasting changes which are evident at genome-wide and candidate gene levels cause aberrant functioning of crucial genes involved in homeostatic responses to environmental challenges.
- A better understanding of the pathways involved in the pathophysiology of mood disorders can result in major advances in the overall management of these recalcitrant conditions.

References

1) Benazzi F. Bipolar II disorder: epidemiology, diagnosis and management. CNS Drugs 2007;21:727–40.
2) Yeh FC, Kao CF, Kuo RH. Explore the features of brain-derived neurotrophic factor in mood disorders. PLoS One 2015;10:e0128605.
3) McNamara RK, Lotrich FE. Elevated immune-inflammatory signaling in mood disorders: a new therapeutic target. Expert Rev Neurother 2012;12:1143–61.
4) Rosenblat JD, Cha DS, Mansur RB, McIntyre RS. Inflammed moods: a review of the interactions between inflammation and mood disorders. Prog Neuropsychopharmacol Biol Psychiatry 2014;53:23–34.
5) Zhang JC, Yao W, Hashimoto K. Brain-derived neurotrophic factor-TrkB signaling in inflammation-related depression and potential therapeutic targets. Curr Neuropharmacol 2016;14:721–31.
6) Grosse L, Ambree O, Jorgens S, Jawahar MC, Singhal G, Stacey D, et al. Cytokine levels in major depression are related to childhood trauma but not to recent stressors. Psychoneuroendocrinology 2016;73:24–31.
7) Rosenblat JD, McIntyre RS. Bipolar disorder and inflammation. Psychiatr Clin North Am 2016;39:125–137.
8) Fernandes BS, Steiner J, Molendijk ML, Dodd S, Nardin P, Gonçalves CA, et al. C-reactive protein concentrations across the mood spectrum in bipolar disorder: a systematic review and meta-analysis. Lancet Psychiatry 2016;3:1147–1156.
9) Goldsmith DR, Rapaport MH, Miller BJ. A meta-analysis of blood cytokine network alterations in psychiatric patients: comparisons between schizophrenia, bipolar disorder and depression. Mol Psychiatry 2016;21:1696–1709.
10) Hestad KA, Tonseth S, Stoen CD, Ueland T, Aukrust P. Raised plasma levels of tumor necrosis factor alpha in patients with depression: normalization during electroconvulsive therapy. J ECT 2003;19:183–188.
11) Tsao CW, Lin YS, Chen CC, Bai CH, Wu SR. Cytokines and serotonin transporter in patients with major depression. Pro Neuropsychopharmacol Biol Psychiatry 2006;30:899–905.
12) Cattaneo A, Gennarelli M, Uher R, Breen G, Farmer A, Aitchison KJ, et al. Candidate genes expression profile associated with antidepressant response in the GENDEP study: differentiating between baseline 'predictors' and 'longitudinal targets'. Neuropsychopharmacology 2013;38:377–385.

13) Mocking RJ, Nap TS, Westerink AM, Assies J, Vaz FM, Koeter MW, et al. Biological profiling of prospective antidepressant response in major depressive disorder: associations with (neuro)inflammation, fatty acid metabolism, and amygdala-reactivity. Psychoneuroendocrinology 2017;79:84–92.

14) Lu S, Peng H, Wang L, Vasish S, Zhang Y, Gao W, et al. Elevated specific cytokines found in major depressive disorder patients with childhood trauma exposure: a cytokine antibody array analysis. Compr Psychiatry 2013;54:953–961.

15) Hartwell KJ, Moran-Santa Maria MM, Twal WO, Shaftman S, DeSantis SM, McRae-Clark AL, et al. Association of elevated cytokines with childhood adversity in a sample of healthy adults. J Psychiatr Res 2013;47:604–610.

16) Miller GE, Cole SW. Clustering of depression and inflammation in adolescents previously exposed to childhood adversity. Biol Psychiatry 2012;72:34–40.

17) Shelton RC, Claiborne J, Sidoryk-Wegrzynowicz M, Reddy R, Aschner M, Lewis DA, et al. Altered expression of genes involved in inflammation and apoptosis in frontal cortex in major depression. Mol Psychiatry 2011;16:751–762.

18) Hung YY, Kang HY, Huang KW, Huang TL. Association between toll-like receptors expression and major depressive disorder. Psychiatry Res 2014;220:283–286.

19) DellaGioia N, Devine L, Pittman B, Hannestad J. Bupropion pre-treatment of endotoxin-induced depressive symptoms. Brain Behav Immun 2013;31:197–204.

20) Dantzer R. Cytokine, sickness behavior, and depression. Immunol Allergy Clin North Am 2009;29:247–264.

21) McCusker RH, Kelley KW. Immune-neural connections: how the immune system's response to infectious agents influences behavior. J Exp Biol 2013; 216:84–98.

22) Miller AH, Haroon E, Raison CL, Felger JC. Cytokine targets in the brain: impact on neurotransmitters and neurocircuits. Depress Anxiety 2013;30:297–306.

23) Myint AM, Kim YK. Network beyond IDO in psychiatric disorders: revisiting neurodegeneration hypothesis. Prog Neuropsychopharmacol Biol Psychiatry 2014;48:304–313.

24) Hashmi AM, Butt Z, Umair M. Is depression an inflammatory condition? A review of available evidence. J Pak Med Assoc 2013;63:899–906.

25) Spijker AT, van Rossum EF. Glucocorticoid sensitivity in mood disorders. Neuroendocrinology 2012;95:179–186.

26) Réus GZ, Fries GR, Stertz L, Badawy M, Passos IC, Barichello T, et al. The role of inflammation and microglia activation in the pathophysiology of psychiatric disorders. Neuroscience 2015;300:141–154.

27) Monje ML, Toda H, Palmer TD. Inflammatory blockade restores adult hippocampal neurogenesis. Science 2003;302:1760–1765.

28) Mattei D, Djodari-Irani A, Hadar R, Pelz A, de Cossío LF, Goetz T, et al. Minocycline rescues decrease in neurogenesis, increase in microglia cytokines and deficits in sensorimotor gating in an animal model of schizophrenia. Brain Behav Immun 2014;38:175–184.

29) Sierra A, Beccari S, Diaz-Aparicio J, Encinas JM, Comeau S, Tremblay ME. Surveillance, phagocytosis, and inflammation: how never-resting microglia influence adult hippocampal neurogenesis. Neural Plast 2014;2014:610343.

30) Kreisel T, Frank MG, Licht T, Reshef R, Ben-Menachem-Zidon O, Barrata MV, et al. Dynamic microglial alterations underlie stress-induced depressive-like behavior and suppressed neurogenesis. Mol Psychiatry 2014;19:699–709.

31) Gebara E, Sultan S, Kocher-Braissant J, Toni N. Adult hippocampal neurogenesis inversely correlates with microglia in conditions of voluntary running and aging. Front Neurosci 2013;7:145.

32) Powell TR, Schalkwyk LC, Hefferman AL, Breen G, Lawrence T, Price T, et al. Tumor necrosis factor and its targets in the inflammatory cytokine pathway are identified as putative transcriptomic biomarkers for escitalopram response. Eur Neuropsychopharmacol 2013;23:1105–1114.

33) Uher R, Tansey KE, Dew T, Maier W, Mors O, Hauser J, et al. An inflammatory biomarker as a differential predictor of outcome of depression treatment with escitalopram and nortriptyline. Am J Psychiatry 2014;171:1278–1286.

34) Uher H, Perroud N, Ng MY, Hauser J, Henigsberg N, Maier W, et al. Genome-wide pharmacogenetics of antidepressant response in the GENDEP project. Am J Psychiatry 2010;167:555–564.

35) Malynn S, Campos-Torres A, Moynagh P, Haase J. The pro-inflammatory cytokine TNF-α regulates the activity and expression of the serotonin transporter (SERT) in astrocytes. Neurochem Res 2013;38:694–704.

36) Haase J, Brown E. Integrating the monoamine, neurotrophin and cytokine hypotheses of depression – a central role for the serotonin transporter? Pharmacol Ther 2015;147:1–11.

37) Yamakawa K, Matsunaga M, Isowa T, Ohira H. Serotonin transporter gene polymorphism modulates inflammatory cytokine responses during acute stress. Sci Rep 2015;5:13852.

38) Ikegame T, Bundo M, Murata Y, Kasai K, Kato T, Iwamoto K. DNA methylation of the BDNF gene and its relevance to psychiatric disorders. J Hum Genet 2013;58:434–438.

39) Karpova NN. Role of BDNF epigenetics in activity-dependent neuronal plasticity. Neuropharmacology 2014;76:709–718.

40) Polyakova M, Stuke K, Schuemberg K, Mueller K, Schoenknecht P, Schroeter ML. BDNF as a biomarker for successful treatment of mood disorders: a systematic & quantitative meta-analysis. J Affect Disord 2015;174:432–440.

41) Molteni R, Cattaneo A, Calabrese F, Macchi F, Olivier JD, Racagni G, et al. Reduced function of the serotonin transporter is associated with decreased expression of BDNF in rodents as well as in humans. Neurobiol Dis 2010;37:747–755.

42) Calabrese F, van der Doelen RH, Guidotti G, Racagni G, Kozicz T, Homberg JR, et al. Exposure to early life stress regulates BDNF expression in SERT mutant rats in an anatomically selective fashion. J Neurochem 2015;132:146–154.

43) Heldt SA, Stanek L, Chhatwal JP, Ressler KJ. Hippocampus-specific deletion of BDNF in adult mice impairs spatial memory and extinction of aversive memories. Mol Psychiatry 2007;12:656–670.

44) Kusumi I, Boku S, Takahashi Y. Psychopharmacology of atypical antipsychotic drugs: from the receptor binding profile to neuroprotection and neurogenesis. Psychiatry Clin Neurosci 2015;69:243–258.

45) Lepack AE, Fuchikami M, Dwyer JM, Banasr M, Duman RS. BDNF release is required for the behavioral actions of ketamine. Int J Neuropsychopharmacol 2015;18:pyu033.

46) Björkholm C, Monteggia LM. BDNF – a key transducer of antidepressant effects. Neuropharmacology 2016;102:72–79.

47) Wang Y, Chang T, Chen YC, Zhang RG, Wang HN, Wu WJ, et al. Quetiapine add-on therapy improves the depressive behaviors and hippocampal neurogenesis in fluoxetine treatment resistant depressive rats. Behav Brain Res 2013;253:206–211.

48) Mandelli L, Petrelli C, Serretti A. The role of specific early trauma in adult depression: a meta-analysis published literature. Childhood trauma and adult depression. Eur Psychiatry 2015;30:665–680.

49) Carr CP, Martins CM, Stingel AM, Lemgruber VB, Juruena MF. The role of early life stress in adult psychiatric disorders: a systematic review according to childhood trauma subtypes. J Nerv Ment Dis 2013;201:1007–1020.

50) Lindert J, von Ehrenstein OS, Grashow R, Gal G, Braehler E, Weisskopf MG. Sexual and physical abuse in childhood is associated with depression and anxiety over the life course: systematic review and meta-analysis. Int J Public Health 2014;59:359–372.

51) Khan A, McCormack HC, Bolger EA, McGreenery CE, Vitaliano G, Polcari A, et al. Childhood maltreatment, depression, and suicidal ideation: critical importance of parental and peer emotional abuse during developmental sensitive periods in males and females. Front Psychiatry 2015;6:42.

52) Cankaya B, Talbot NL, Ward EA, Duberstein PR. Parental sexual abuse and suicidal behavior among women with major depressive disorder. Can J Psychiatry 2012;57:45–51.

53) Zeugmann S, Buehrsch N, Bajbouj M, Heuser I, Anghelescu I, Quante A. Childhood maltreatment and adult proinflammatory status in patients with major depression. Psychiatr Danub 2013;25:227–235.

54) Danese A, Moffitt TE, Pariante CM, Ambler A, Poulton R, Caspi A. Elevated inflammation levels in depressed adults with a history of childhood maltreatment. Arch Gen Psychiatry 2008;65:409–415.

55) Coelho R, Viola TW, Walss-Bass C, Brietzke E, Grassi-Oliveira R. Childhood maltreatment and inflammatory markers: a systematic review. Acta Psychiatr Scand 2014;129:180–192.

56) Pace TW, Mletzko TC, Alagbe O, Musselman DL, Nemeroff CB, Miller AH, Heim CM. Increased stress-induced inflammatory responses in male patients with major depression and increased early life stress. Am J Psychiatry 2006;163:1630–1633.

57) Miller G, Chen E. Unfavorable socioeconomic conditions in early life presage expression of proinflammatory phenotype in adolescence. Psychosom Med 2007;69:402–409.

58) Rohleder N, Wolf JM, Wolf OT. Glucocorticoid sensitivity of cognitive and inflammatory processes in depression and posttraumatic stress disorder. Neurosci Biobehav Rev 2010;35:104–114.

59) Janusek LW, Tell D, Gaylord-Harden N, Mathews HL. Relationship of childhood adversity and neighborhood violence to a proinflammatory phenotype in emerging adult African American men: an epigenetic link. Brain Behav Immun 2017;60:126–135.

60) Sominsky L, Fuller EA, Bondarenko E, Ong LK, Averell L, Nalivaiko E, et al. Functional programming of the autonomic nervous system by early life immune exposure: implications for anxiety. PLoS One 2013;8:e57700.

61) Walker AK, Nakamura T, Hodgson DM. Neonatal lipopolysaccharide exposure alters responses to stress in adulthood in Wistar rats. Stress 2010;13:506–515.

62) Doherty TS, Forster A, Roth TL. Global and gene-specific DNA methylation alterations in the adolescent amygdala and hippocampus in an animal model of caregiver maltreatment. Behav Brain Res 2016;298:55–61.

63) Blaze J, Scheuing L, Roth TL. Differential methylation of genes in the medial prefrontal cortex of developing and adult rats following exposure to maltreatment or nurturing care during infancy. Dev Neurosci 2013;35:306–316.

64) Roceri M, Cirulli F, Pessina C, Peretto P, Racagni G, Riva MA. Postnatal repeated maternal deprivation produces age-dependent changes of brain-derived neurotrophic factor expression in selected brain regions. Biol Psychiatry 2004;55:708–714.

65) Luoni A, Berry A, Calabrese F, Capoccia S, Bellisario V, Gass P, et al. Delayed BDNF alterations in the prefrontal cortex of rats exposed to prenatal stress: preventive effect of lurasidone treatment during adolescence. Eur Neuropsychopharmacol 2014;24:986–995.

66) Orefice LL, Waterhouse EG, Partridge JG, Lalchandani RR, Vicini S, Xu B. Distinct roles for somatically and dendritically synthesized brain-derived neurotrophic factor in morphogenesis of dendritic spines. J Neurosci 2013;33:11618–11632.

67) Orefice LL, Shih CC, Xu H, Waterhouse EG, Xu B. Control of spine maturation and pruning through proBDNF synthesized and released in dendrites. Mol Cell Neurosci 2016;71:66–79.

68) Lau AG, Irier HA, Gu J, Tian D, Ku L, Liu G, et al. Distinct 3'UTRs differentially regulate activity-dependent translation of brain-derived neurotrophic factor (BDNF). Proc Natl Acad Sci USA 2010;107:15945–15950.

69) Kolb B, Gibb R. Plasticity in the prefrontal cortex of adult rats. Front Cell Neurosci 2015;9:15.

70) Belnoue L, Grosjean N, Ladeveze E, Abrous DN, Koehl M. Prenatal stress inhibits hippocampal neurogenesis but spares olfactory bulb neurogenesis. PLoS One 2013;8:e72972.

71) Schwabe L, Bohbot VD, Wolf OT. Prenatal stress changes learning strategies in adulthood. Hippocampus 2012;22:2136–2143.

72) Ventriglio A, Gentile A, Baldessarini RJ, Bellomo A. Early-life stress and psychiatric disorders: epidemiology, neurobiology and innovative pharmacological targets. Curr Pharm Des 2015;21:1379–1387.

73) Oomen CA, Soeters H, Audureau N, Vermunt L, van Hasselt FN, Manders EM, et al. Early maternal deprivation affects dentate gyrus structure and emotional learning in adult female rats. Psychopharmacology (Berl) 2011;214:249–260.

74) Lajud N, Roque A, Cajero M, Gutiérrez-Ospina G, Torner L. Periodic maternal separation decreases hippocampal neurogenesis without affecting basal corticosterone during the stress hyporesponsive period, but alters HPA axis and coping behavior in adulthood. Psychoneuroendocrinology 2012;37:410–420.

75) Calabrese F, Luoni A, Guidotti G, Racagni G, Fumagalli F, Riva MA. Modulation of neuronal plasticity following chronic concomitant administration of the novel antipsychotic lurasidone with the mood stabilizer valproic acid. Psychopharmacology (Berl) 2013;226:101–112.

76) Nestler EJ. Transgenerational epigenetic contributions to stress responses: fact or fiction? PLoS Biol 2016;14:e1002426.

77) Vialou V, Feng J, Robison AJ, Nestler EJ. Epigenetic mechanisms of depression and antidepressant action. Annu Rev Pharmacol Toxicol 2013;53:59–87.

78) Babenko O, Kovalchuk I, Metz GA. Stress-induced perinatal and transgenerational epigenetic programming of brain and mental health. Neurosci Biobehav Rev 2015;48:70–91.

79) Bockmühl Y, Patchev AV, Madejska A, Hoffmann A, Sousa JC, Sousa N, et al. Methylation at the CpG island shore region upregulates Nr3c1 promoter activity after early-life stress. Epigenetics 2015;10:247–257.

80) Massart R, Mongeau R, Lanfumey L. Beyond the monoaminergic hypothesis: neuroplasticity and epigenetic changes in a transgenic mouse model of depression. Philos Trans R Soc Lond B Biol Sci 2012;367:2485–2494.

81) Murgatroyd C, Spengler D. Polycomb binding preceded early-life stress responsive DNA methylation at the Avp enhancer. PLoS One 2014;9:e90277.

82) McGowan PO, Sasaki A, D'Alessio AC, Dymov S, Labonte B, Szyf M, et al. Epigenetic regulation of the glucocorticoid receptor in human brain associates with childhood abuse. Nat Neurosci 2009;12:342–348.

83) Labonte B, Yerko V, Gross J, Mechawar N, Meaney MJ, Szyf M, et al. Differential glucocorticoid receptor exon 1(B), 1(C), and 1(H) expression and methylation in suicide completers with a history of childhood abuse. Biol Psychiatry 2012;72:41–48.

84) Mitchelmore C, Gede L. Brain Derived Neurotrophic Factor: epigenetic regulation in psychiatric disorders. Brain Res 2014;1586:162–172.

85) Tsankova NM, Berton O, Renthal W, Kumar A, Neve RL, Nestler EJ. Sustained hippocampal chromatin regulation in a mouse model of depression and antidepressant action. Nat Neurosci 2006;9:519–525.

86) Molteni R, Cattaneo A, Calabrese F, Macchi F, Olivier JD, Racagni G, et al. Reduced function of the serotonin transporter is associated with decreased expression of BDNF in rodents as well as in humans. Neurobiol Dis 2010;37:747–755.

87) Keller S, Sarchiapone M, Zarrilli F, Videtic A, Ferraro A, Carli V, et al. Increased BDNF promoter methylation in the Wernicke area of suicide subjects. Arch Gen Psychiatry 2010;67:258–267.

88) Roth TL, Lubin FD, Funk AJ, Sweatt JD. Lasting epigenetic influence of early-life adversity on the BDNF gene. Biol Psychiatry 2009;65:760–769.

89) Smith AK, Kilaru V, Klengel T, Mercer KB, Bradley B, Conneely KN, et al. DNA extracted from saliva for methylation studies of psychiatric traits: evidence tissue specificity and relatedness to brain. Am J Med Genet B Neuropsychiatr Genet 2015;168B:36–44.

90) Kundakovic M, Gudsnuk K, Herbstman JB, Tang D, Perera FP, Champagne FA. DNA methylation of BDNF as a biomarker of early-life adversity. Proc Natl Acad Sci U S A 2015;112:6807–6813.

91) Klengel T, Pape J, Binder EB, Mehta D. The role of DNA methylation in stress-related psychiatric disorders. Neuropharmacology 2014;80:115–132.

92) Provençal N, Suderman MJ, Guillemin C, Massart R, Ruggiero A, Wang D, et al. The signature of maternal rearing in the methylome in rhesus macaque prefrontal cortex and T cells. J Neurosci 2012;32:15626–15642.

93) Provencal N, Binder EB. The neurobiological effects of stress as contributors to psychiatric disorders: focus on epigenetics. Curr Opin Neurobiol 2015;30:31–37.

94) Ligthart S, Marzi C, Aslibekyan S, Mendelson MM, Conneely KN, Tanaka T, et al. DNA methylation signatures of chronic low-grade inflammation are associated with complex diseases. Genome Biol 2016;17:255.

5   Neurobiology of Mood Disorders
The Circadian Connection

Introduction

Severe mood disturbances represented by unipolar depression and bipolar disorder (BD) have a common theme: the disruption of the 24-hour sleep–wake cycle. This disturbance is essentially present in mood episodes and recognized by both the Diagnostic and Statistical Manual of Mental Disorders – 5th Edition (DSM-5) and the International Classification of Diseases – 10th Revision (ICD-10) as required criteria for the purpose of diagnosis.[1] Early morning wakening is a characteristic symptom of melancholic depression, wherein the patient wakes up after only a few hours of sleep and is unable to resume sleep for the rest of the night. While depression is marked by a reduction in total sleep duration, manic patients with boundless energy feel rested after only a few hours of sleep and continue with their schedules uninterrupted. Coupled with this phenomenon are other manifestations such as diurnal mood variations, and changes in appetite and energy levels, which signify a key disturbance in the circadian system.[2] Whereas severe affective episodes are marked by an extreme disruption in the daily cycle, all active treatments, which include medications, chronobiological measures and psychotherapies, restore the circadian rhythm. In essence, remission of mood episodes is preceded by a realignment of the sleep–wake cycle and an interruption in the latter is the harbinger of an imminent relapse.[3]

The Social Zeitgeber (German for "time giver") Theory of mood disorders was put forth in the late 1980s, proposing that stressful life events cause alterations in the sleep–wake schedule which subsequently modify molecular and cellular rhythms in susceptible individuals, leading to mood-related episodes.[4] However, the mechanisms by which circadian rhythm disturbances might cause fluctuations in affective states have not been fully elucidated. Over the years, several theories have been put forward to explain the development of mood disorders. While the circadian system is best known for its part in regulating the timing of sleep, and certainly significant sleep changes like shift work and irregular schedules can precipitate or aggravate mood-related problems, it is now becoming clear that the clock machinery is intricately involved in the molecular and cellular control of a wide range of processes which are

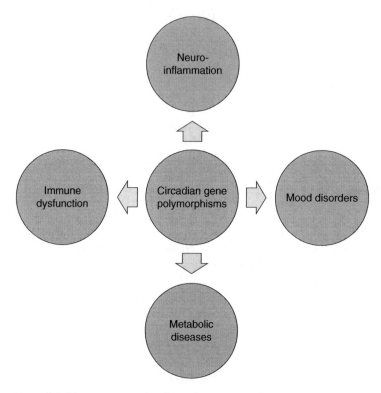

Figure 5.1 The pervasive role of circadian genes in disease processes

Circadian genes are expressed throughout the body and the brain, where they participate in essential physiological functions. Alterations in the DNA sequence and/or epigenetic modifications can result in aberrant functioning of these genes, with pathogenic consequences, such as the development of neuropsychiatric disorders and systemic diseases. These conditions are exemplified by mood disorders, metabolic syndrome, dysfunctional immunity and a variety of cancers.

postulated to trigger affective episodes.[5] A better knowledge of these mechanisms can enhance our understanding of mood disorders in general, and the ensuing multifarious complications in particular. In this vein, Figure 5.1 is helpful in understanding the involvement of circadian gene polymorphisms in the development of a wide range of diseases.

Mood Disorders and the Circadian System

The Master Circadian Oscillator

The control of the daily rhythms is regulated from a small assembly of neurons located in the suprachiasmatic nucleus (SCN) of the hypothalamus which receives light input through a direct connection, the retinohypothalamic tract. The SCN then sends signals via direct and indirect projections throughout the brain. It also coordinates the timing of the release of multiple peptides and hormones including melatonin, which promotes sleep onset. Intriguingly, the SCN appears to control the timing of rhythms in the periphery via alterations in body temperature which serve as a universal cue to entrain multiple organ systems to the light–dark cycle.[6] The expression of clock-controlled genes regulates rhythmic functions including the sleep–wake cycle, feeding behavior, release of hormones and metabolic regulation. The clock genes are widely expressed throughout the cells of the peripheral organs such as the liver, endocrine tissues, heart, skeletal muscles, etc., where these participate in the performance of essential functions, vital for survival. Indeed, it is now recognized that 70% of the mammalian genome is rhythmic in nature and all major bodily functions are regulated in a circadian manner.[7]

The Core Molecular Clock

The SCN neurons house the circadian molecular hub, while the clock itself is composed of a series of transcriptional and translational feedback loops that result in the rhythmic expression of clock genes on a timescale of just over 24 hours. In the primary feedback loop, the transcription factors, Circadian Locomotor Output Cycles Kaput (CLOCK) and Brain and Muscle Arnt-Like protein 1 (BMAL1), heterodimerize and bind to E-box containing sequences in a number of genes including the three Period (PER) genes (PER1, PER2 and PER3) and two Cryptochrome (CRY) genes (CRY1 and CRY2). Over time PER and CRY proteins dimerize in the cytosol and are shuttled back into the nucleus where CRY proteins can directly inhibit the activity of CLOCK and BMAL1. In addition to this feedback loop, the CLOCK and BMAL1 proteins regulate the expression of Rev-erbα and ROR (retinoic acid-related orphan nuclear receptors) which in turn can repress or activate BMAL1 transcription respectively, through action at the Rev-Erb/ROR response element in the promoter. There are several key proteins which regulate the timing of the molecular clock through phosphorylation, sumoylation and other mechanisms. The enzymes, casein kinases, phosphorylate the PER, CRY and BMAL1 proteins altering their stability and nuclear entry; glycogen synthase kinase 3 beta (GSK3β) also phosphorylates the PER2 protein facilitating its nuclear entry.[8] As alluded to above many controlling kinases, phosphatases and secondary feedback loops act on the molecular clock, contributing to great intricacy to the circadian apparatus. Significantly, circadian transcription factors are involved in the regulation and functioning of several other clock-controlled genes, which partake in a whole range of homeostatic actions in every body system. As will become clear in the ensuing sections, these sub-cellular mechanisms regulate the key physiological functions of the body in a circadian fashion.

Human and Animal Genetic Studies

More than 50 genetic studies in humans have incriminated clock genes in psychiatric diseases. These have used a variety of approaches, e.g., candidate genes, genome-wide association studies, copy number variants and transcriptomics/proteomics. It can be argued that circadian rhythm anomalies are the cause rather than the effect of mood disruptions, yet possibly one aggravates the other.[9]

In this respect, rodent studies have been very helpful in explaining the role of circadian genes in depression and anxiety-like behaviors. Mice with an induced mutation in the CLOCK gene, which creates a protein with dominant-negative function (ClockΔ19), have a behavioral profile which is reminiscent of BD, particularly in the manic state. When these animals are given the classical mood stabilizer, lithium, the bulk of their behavioral responses are normalized towards those of wild-type mice.[10]

Mice engineered bearing other circadian gene mutations exhibit comparable behavioral phenotypes. These include transgenic mice overexpressing GSK3β and those with a mutation in F-box protein 3 (Fbxl3, a protein that targets CRY for degradation). Sirtuin 1 (SIRT1) is a histone deacetylase which antagonizes the actions of transcription factors CLOCK and BMAL1. SIRT1 knockout mice also have a decrease in anxiety-like behavior at baseline, and lowered depression-related behavior following chronic social defeat paradigm. Overexpression of SIRT1 leads to the opposite effect. SIRT1 knockout should lead to increased CLOCK activity yet the mutant mouse has a similar manic-like phenotype, suggesting that perhaps any circadian gene mutation will lead to the same behavioral profile.[11] However, while PER2 knockout mice also have reduced immobility in the Porsolt's forced swim test, mice with mutations in both PER1 and PER2 (double mutants) have a normal locomotor response in the novelty seeking test, and an increase in anxiety-related behavior which is the opposite of what is observed in the ClockΔ19 and other mutant mice.[12] Therefore, the observed rodent behavior in a variety of investigational conditions suggests that circadian genes have some specificity in their function and the same phenotype is not produced with the mutation of any circadian factor. Of course, some of these proteins are involved in other processes besides daily rhythm regulation and it is conceivable that the mood and anxiety-related behavioral phenotypes are due to alterations in other physiological systems.

The Neurobiology of the Circadian System

Monoamine Signaling in Mood Disorders

The modern era of psychopharmacology was ushered in the 1950s with the discovery of medications that possessed a tricyclic structure, e.g., chlorpromazine, imipramine and amitriptyline. Soon afterwards it was found that these compounds effected monoamine transmission in the brain by a variety of mechanisms, for example by blocking the synaptic transporters or antagonizing the postsynaptic receptors, and this was their initial pharmacodynamic action. Even after the passage of several decades, the modern psychotherapeutic agents are still based on the same principle and all current medications act by manipulating the monoamine neurotransmitters. For example, the major class of antidepressant drugs used now are selective serotonin reuptake inhibitors (SSRIs). Multiple human functional imaging studies using PET, SPECT and fMRI have also found alterations in these systems in subjects with mood disorders.[13] Administration of the antidepressant, agomelatine (a melatonin receptor agonist and weak 5-HT2C receptor antagonist), leads to increases in monoaminergic neuronal activity which can be blocked with the melatonergic antagonist S22153. These results point to a modulatory role for the pineal hormone, melatonin, in monoaminergic activity, linking the circadian and monoamine systems.[14]

Rodent studies employing novel research methodologies like optogenetics have confirmed the importance of the monoaminergic circuitry in mood, reward and anxiety-related behavior. Some results are intriguing in that the stimulation of dopamine neurons in the ventral tegmental area (VTA) can lead to both a pro-depressive and antidepressive response in certain chronic stress paradigms, with great importance for understanding such phenomena as rapid cycling, mood switching and mixed states.[15] It is known that serotonin, norepinephrine and dopamine all have a circadian rhythm in their synthesis, release and receptors. Since these systems are clearly involved in arousal, motivation and reward, it would be of evolutionary value for these circuits to have a diurnal rhythm so that activities directly linked to survival are not in chronological disagreement with the internal drive to sleep. Some of the rhythms in these circuits arise from projections from the SCN. All of these monoamine neuronal populations also express circadian genes which directly regulate expression of genes involved in neurotransmitter synthesis and release. One example is monoamine oxidase A (MAOA), a gene important in monoaminergic metabolism, which is a direct transcriptional target of the clock proteins NPAS2, BMAL1 and PER2 in the striatum.[16]

PER2 mutant mice have increased dopamine levels and altered neuronal activity in the striatum, which may explain some of their abnormal behavioral phenotypes in measures of mood, reward and anxiety. In response to chronic stress, PER1 and PER2 mRNA levels are altered in the nucleus accumbens (NAc). Furthermore, selective knock-down of both PER1 and PER2 via RNA interference in the NAc is adequate to produce an increase in anxiety-like behavior, suggesting prominent roles for the PER genes in this region.[17] ClockΔ19 mutant mice have increased dopamine synthesis and increased dopaminergic activity. Moreover, they have an increase in tyrosine hydroxylase (TH) expression in the VTA. Continued lithium treatment restores normal levels of VTA dopaminergic activity to the ClockΔ19 mutants suggesting that dopamine overactivity may underlie the manic-like behavior. The regulation of TH expression and dopamine levels by CLOCK seems to be evolutionarily conserved as fruit flies which carry a mutation in the CLOCK gene have increased TH levels and increased dopamine synthesis.[18] Many, but not all, of the manic-like phenotypes of the ClockΔ19 mice are rescued by expression of a functional CLOCK protein, precisely in the VTA. Remarkably, knock-down of CLOCK expression only in the VTA of otherwise wild-type mice leads to a "mixed state" in which mice are less anxious and hyperactive, but express more depressive-like behaviors. This has translational significance, in view of the fact that mood disorder patients cycle through periods of depression, mania and mixed states.[19] Hence, circadian genes appear to have a direct role in the VTA and there are likely other monoaminergic regions which are important in the regulation of anxiety and mood-related behavior. Indisputably, this area of research is crucial in understanding the connections that link disrupted circadian rhythms to mood disorders and will certainly be the focus of future studies.

The CLOCK Proteins and the Immune-Inflammatory System

Several lines of evidence have linked immune-inflammatory abnormalities with mood disorders. For instance, there is an increased incidence of depression in such medical conditions as rheumatoid arthritis, inflammatory bowel disease and asthma. Many patients who are given cytokine therapy, like peg-interferon, for hepatitis C develop recurrent depressive episodes, and increased levels of proinflammatory markers like C-reactive protein are found in patients with mood disorders. Therefore, a neuroinflammatory hypothesis has been proposed to elucidate the development of major mood disorders, and is gaining precedence with accumulating research evidence.[20] In humans and animal models, proinflammatory cytokines can themselves induce a syndrome resembling depression with feelings of anhedonia, psychomotor slowing and fatigue. In the rodent hippocampus, proinflammatory cytokines lead to reduced neurogenesis, decreased synaptic plasticity, and less long-term potentiation, which is similar to effects seen with chronic stress models of depression.[21] Additionally, the reduction in neurogenesis and abnormal behaviors produced in response to stress can be blocked with inhibitors of the transcription factor nuclear factor-κB (NF-κB). Proinflammatory cytokines can also impact monoamine signaling leading to reductions in 5-HT release, as well as altered HPA axis function in animal models, linking several systems that are crucial to the pathogenesis of mood disorders.[22]

Circadian rhythm disruption in humans and animal models leads to an increase in proinflammatory cytokines including interleukin-6 (IL-6), IL-1β and tumor necrosis factor-alpha (TNF-α). In turn, these inflammatory mediators alter the sleep–wake cycle and circadian gene expression via NF-κB signaling pathways. Several studies have found that a lipopolysaccharide-induced immune challenge leads to a depressive-like phenotype in rodents and also alters circadian gene expression and SCN activity.[23] Intriguingly, a central infusion of IL-1β causes a significant phase delay in locomotor rhythms, a state often associated with an increased risk for depression in animal experiments. Constant darkness (for four weeks) in rodents leads to both increased depression-like behavior and elevated levels of plasma IL-6 and hippocampal IL-1 receptor, type 1. In addition, mice with a deletion of IL-6 (a target gene of

NF-κB) do not develop depression-like behavior in constant darkness, suggesting a prominent role for NF-κB signaling and cytokine induction in the development of depression-like behavior following diurnal rhythm disruption.[24] Recently, it was discovered that the CLOCK protein interacts directly with NF-κB to activate transcription at NF-κB responsive promoters. Furthermore, activation of NF-κB in response to immunological stimuli is reduced in cells which lack the CLOCK protein. Interestingly, RORα inhibits NF-κB function by inducing a protein that antagonizes NF-κB signaling. Hence, there appears to be complex bidirectional cross talk between the circadian and immune systems.[25] Accordingly, a scenario could be proposed in which genetic or environmental disruptions of circadian rhythms lead to a proinflammatory response in the brain which alters monoamine signaling, SCN function and hippocampal neuroplasticity, ultimately leading to a depression-like state.[26] There is no doubt that further research would clarify the mechanisms connecting circadian rhythm disturbances, immune-inflammatory abnormalities and the development of mood disorders.

Regulation of the Hypothalamic–Pituitary–Adrenal Axis

Glucocorticoids (cortisol in humans, corticosterone in lower species like rodents) are pleiotropic adrenal steroid hormones which participate in numerous physiological functions including metabolism and homeostasis. These are also closely involved in the response to stress via the activation of the HPA axis. Glucocorticoids have a strong circadian rhythm in expression and peak in levels just prior to the onset of awakening. Interestingly, this is the exact opposite of the melatonin rhythm, since it peaks in the late evening and ebbs by the morning. The glucocorticoid receptor (GR) is the main mediator of the actions of cortisol, and CRY proteins interact with GR in a ligand-dependent fashion leading to rhythmic repression in its activity. Furthermore, CLOCK directly acetylates GR leading to decreased sensitivity to glucocorticoids in the morning and increased sensitivity at night when acetylation is reversed.[27]

Severe mood episodes are characterized by the loss of the diurnal variation of cortisol response, wherein its levels remain elevated in the evening with flattening of the cortisol curve. Persistent hypercortisolemia is an ominous sign since it represents non-remission of the affective episode, treatment resistance and increased likelihood of suicidal behavior. This phenomenon has been documented in melancholic depression, psychotic mood episodes and patients with high levels of suicidality.[28] It can be assumed that the more severe the disruption in the glucocorticoid rhythm, the greater the intensity of the mood disturbance and the higher the risk to the patient. Conversely, there is evidence to suggest that antidepressant treatment helps in restoring the HPA axis function via the serotonergic system. Hence, it is fair to propose that the restoration of cortisol rhythm in mood disorder patients is beneficial to mood stabilization. Additionally, the direct regulation of GR expression and activity by circadian genes is extremely important in mediating the response to chronic stress.[29]

The Circadian Control of Metabolism

Circadian rhythms in the liver, stomach, adipose tissue and gut are robust, leading to distinct 24-hour cycles in metabolic functions. Peptides involved in metabolism and feeding like ghrelin, orexin, leptin and cholecystokinin (CCK) exhibit a marked circadian rhythm in expression. In human blood samples, leptin is increased during the night, orexin levels are elevated during the day and ghrelin and CCK are high prior to meals and at night.[30] Both leptin and ghrelin signal through orexin neurons in the brain, enhancing wakefulness when stimulated by ghrelin and promoting sleep when inhibited by leptin. In narcolepsy, a condition in which individuals experience sudden sleep bouts, there is dysfunction of the orexin system, linking regulation of feeding and sleep to a small population of hypothalamic neurons. CCK is more widely expressed throughout the brain and gut including high levels of expression in GABAergic interneurons of the prefrontal cortex, dopaminergic neurons of the VTA, and the shell of the SCN.[31] These peptides and others involved in feeding behaviors are out of sync in the ClockΔ19 mice, demonstrating that their expression is regulated by the core molecular clock. Furthermore, ClockΔ19 mice gain weight rapidly on a high fat diet and display many features of obesity and the metabolic syndrome.[32]

Both ghrelin and leptin from the periphery modulate reward-related circuits in the brain. Moreover, ghrelin (Ghr −/−) knockout mice are more anxious after acute restraint stress which is likely due to an aberration in the normal glucocorticoid feedback response in this situation.[33] Ghrelin receptor-null mice also show a greater response in the chronic social defeat stress paradigm compared to wild-type mice. Interestingly, chronic social defeat stress produces long-lasting disruptions in body temperature rhythms and in the diurnal variations of plasma ghrelin and leptin. Thus proper daily rhythms in ghrelin and leptin signaling may be important in mood regulation.[34]

Many studies have found a prominent role for CCK in the regulation of anxiety-related and mood-related behavior. Increased CCK or CCK receptor agonists are generally associated with heightened anxiety. In turn, CCK receptor antagonists have antidepressant-like properties in acute rodent measures of behavioral despair. Moreover, chronic blockade of CCK receptors prevents HPA axis hyperactivity, reduction of hippocampal volume and cell proliferation and decreases sucrose intake normally evoked by repeated social defeat stress.[35] CCK is co-released with dopamine in the NAc and acts to silence dopamine neurons in the VTA. CCK has a strong circadian rhythm in expression in the VTA and is a direct transcriptional target of CLOCK in this region. ClockΔ19 mice have very low levels of CCK in the VTA and increased dopaminergic activity. In a recent study it was demonstrated that treatment with lithium restores CCK expression to wild-type levels in the ClockΔ19 mice through changes in chromatin structure at the CCK promoter.[36] Moreover, CCK knock-down in the VTA is sufficient to recapitulate many of the manic-like behaviors of the ClockΔ19 mice. Interestingly, CCK knock-down in the basolateral amygdala has anxiolytic and antidepressant effects in mice suggesting that it is involved in modulating activity within multiple limbic regions.

The abovementioned animal studies are sufficient to show the interaction of circadian genes, metabolic peptides and behavior. The relationships between affective disorders and metabolic abnormalities is well recognized and it is interesting to note that the daily rhythm, which is fundamentally disturbed in mood disorder patients, could have an important role in the pathogenesis of metabolic anomalies. Furthermore, there is unquestionably a requirement for more studies which examine the metabolic and mood-related effects that come with therapeutic treatments which improve sleep and circadian rhythms. Finally, the mechanisms mediating disrupted rhythms in metabolic dysfunctions and the underlying neurobiological substrates have yet to be fully explored in people with various mood disturbances.[37]

Oxidative Stress and the Circadian System

Mitochondria are the organelles in which oxidative phosphorylation of substrates takes place and adenosine triphosphate (ATP) is generated, which is used in the performance of essential cellular functions. A mitochondrial dysfunction hypothesis of psychiatric disorders, particularly BD, has been offered based on the following findings[38]:

1) Abnormalities in mitochondrial morphology, cellular localization and mitochondrial DNA sequences are found in postmortem brain samples from bipolar subjects.
2) Patients with BD have increased bursts of energy, racing thoughts, flight of ideas and overactivity that are likely due to augmented metabolism.
3) Conversely, patients with mitochondrial diseases often have comorbid mood disorders.
4) Bipolar subjects exhibit altered energy metabolism in the brain, as assessed by functional neuroimaging, and abnormal respiratory chain activity in peripheral cells resembling patients with mitochondrial disorders.

BD is also related to increased dendritic loss and neuronal death. On the other hand, anti-apoptotic and neuroprotective proteins like Bcl-2 are robustly induced by mood stabilizing medications. Intriguingly, mice with forebrain-specific mitochondrial DNA mutations have behaviors that resemble human mania including altered circadian rhythms. The mitochondria supply most of the cell's ATP and are involved in controlling the redox state of the cell.

Nicotinamide cofactors NADPH/NADP+ and NADH/NAD+ have recently been identified as essential partners of CLOCK, NPAS2 and SIRT1, providing a direct link between the redox state of the cell and circadian rhythms.[39] Moreover, CLOCK/BMAL1 directly regulate the expression of nicotinamide phosphoribosyltransferase in a circadian fashion which then determines the availability of NAD+ in the cell over 24 hours.

Another measure of cellular metabolism is the ratio of AMP and ATP. An important sensor of the AMP/ATP ratio is adenosine monophosphate-dependent protein kinase (AMPK) which is activated upon binding to AMP. AMPK is stimulated in neurons in response to metabolic or ischemic stressors and elicits compensatory responses. AMPK phosphorylates casein kinase 1 epsilon which enhances phosphorylation of PER2, again directly pairing cellular metabolism to the circadian system.[40] Moreover, the mitochondrial biogenesis stimulator, "peroxisome proliferator-activated receptor gamma coactivator 1-α", directly regulates expression of BMAL1 and Rev-erbα and is necessary for circadian pacemaker function.[41] The eventual results of metabolic dysfunction in neurons are oxidative stress, generation of reactive oxygen species and apoptosis. Therefore, given the close link between the circadian system and redox signaling, it seems reasonable to speculate that circadian rhythm disruption might lead to the accumulation of damaging free radicals and enhanced neuronal apoptosis. In fact the apoptotic genes, Wnt10, β-catenin, Dishevelled2 and transcription factor 3 promoters, are all bound by BMAL1, and Wnt pathway signaling is attenuated when BMAL1 levels are reduced. Aberrant Wnt and GSK3 signaling is implicated in mood disorders and there is emerging evidence to demonstrate that the circadian system is intimately involved in the regulation of these pathways.[42]

It is also interesting to note that many of the genes involved in apoptosis are also involved in neuroplasticity. Thus the pharmacodynamic response to antidepressant or mood stabilizing medications enhancing new cell formation in the neurogenic niche of the brain may involve these same pathways directly regulated by the circadian system.[43] Indeed, as major mood disorders do not seem to be generally associated with severe neurodegeneration, the influence of cellular stress-related pathways are likely much more subtle and perhaps alter plasticity and dendritic complexity, rather than causing direct neuronal death.

The Circadian Rhythm and Neurogenesis

The neurogenic hypothesis of mood disorders originates from animal studies demonstrating that chronic stress and behavioral models of depression reduce hippocampal neurogenesis, while psychotropic medications enhance neurogenesis. Whereas the process of neurogenesis varies greatly over the circadian cycle, there is a functional link between the expression of PER2 and the regulation of cell proliferation and apoptosis in the dentate gyrus (DG) of the hippocampus.[44] Continuing disruption in circadian rhythms via weekly phase shifts inhibits hippocampal neurogenesis, and the degree of this reduction is contingent on the direction and duration of the shifts.[45] Physiological variations in corticosterone can help regulate the rhythmic expression of PER1 in the DG. Moreover, regular diurnal corticosterone rhythm is necessary for the proliferation of progenitor cells in the DG in response to the SSRI, fluoxetine. Flattening of the diurnal corticosterone rhythm in rats also prevents the stimulating action of L-NAME (a nitric oxide synthase inhibitor) on progenitor cell proliferation in the DG as well as brain-derived neurotrophic factor (BDNF) and tyrosine receptor kinase B (TrkB) expression.[46] BDNF and its receptor, TrkB, have been shown in several studies to be important in the actions of psychotropic medications and both have a strong circadian rhythm in expression in the hippocampus. In rodent models, BDNF loses its effects on cell proliferation rates in the absence of a daily rhythm in corticosterone. These results indicate that the diurnal rhythm of corticosterone regulates the stimulating action of psychopharmacological agents on neurogenesis and BDNF signaling in the DG. As such, it will be important in future studies to determine the impact of circadian gene mutations on neurogenesis and TrkB signaling following psychotropic drug treatment. In conclusion, it can be inferred from the evidence presented that the formation and integration of new neurons is highly dependent on a normal diurnal rhythm, as glucocorticoids and neurotrophins cannot carry out their roles without a normal circadian cycle.[47]

Figure 5.2 provides a schematic rendition of the disturbance in core biological processes caused by a disrupted circadian clock, with pathogenic consequences to different organ systems of the body.

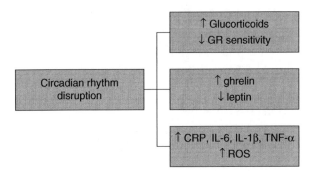

Figure 5.2 Biological effects of the disruption in circadian rhythms

In affective episodes, the daily rhythm is disrupted with disturbances in the sleep–wake cycle, irregular meal times and lop-sided social schedules. These aberrations result in numerous detrimental physiological consequences effecting all systems of the body. For instance, impaired stress reaction manifests as hypercortisolemia, insensitivity of the glucocorticoid receptor (GR) and abnormal response of the HPA axis. Metabolic peptides are out of sync resulting in insulin resistance, glucose intolerance and the metabolic syndrome. Immune function is compromised with raised C-reactive protein (CRP) and proinflammatory cytokines, ultimately contributing to neuroinflammation and cardiovascular disorders, among other abnormalities. Generation of reactive oxygen species (ROS) further enhances neuroinflammation with increased apoptosis of neurons and decreased neurogenesis.

Conclusion

Indeed, research in the past few decades has unraveled the importance of the circadian system in the regulation of mood through a variety of mechanisms. As noted by the psychiatrists in the mid-twentieth century, abnormalities in daily rhythm are central to major mood disorders. It is mainly through animal research that the underlying neurobiology of this association is being clarified. For instance, it is now known that circadian genes are not only found in the SCN, but rather are expressed throughout the brain and the body. The circadian genes are clearly involved in the regulation of immune function, monoamine neurotransmission, neurogenesis, endocrine homeostasis and control of metabolism. It is very likely that the disruption of the circadian rhythm alters mood through multiple biological pathways. Indeed, all of these systems feed into one another and interact at multiple levels. The circadian system has a pervasive role in physiological functioning and its disruption can manifest as neuropsychiatric disturbances and somatic ailments. This system of overarching significance is now being targeted for drug development in the hopes of

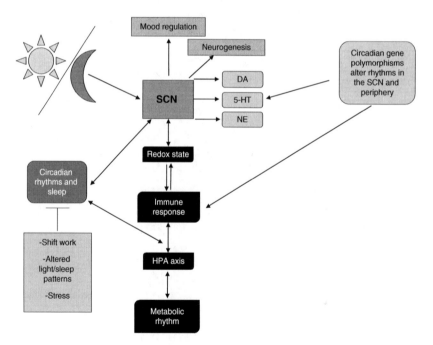

Figure 5.3 The relationship between mood regulation and the circadian system

The circadian clock affects several systems and pathways which are supposedly the cause of mood disorders. In the majority of patients there are shared aberrant connections which lead to dysregulated daily oscillations. Circadian gene mutations possibly make a person more susceptible to affective disturbances and these are worsened by environmental variations in the daily timetable.

5-HT – 5-hydroxytryptamine; DA – dopamine; HPA axis – hypothalamic–pituitary–adrenal axis; NE – norepinephrine; SCN – suprachiasmatic nucleus treating a number of diseases including cancer, obesity, sleep disorders and diabetes. It is likely that such future developments would also be beneficial for the treatment of mood disorders.

Figure 5.3 puts into perspective the interacting mechanisms underlying mood disorders from the standpoint of circadian gene polymorphisms with downstream effects throughout the brain and the body.

Summary Points

- Circadian disturbance is essentially present in all types of mood episodes.
- The molecular machinery of the chronobiological clock is highly intricate and composed of several transcription factors, genes and proteins which are regulated by key enzymes of the kinome.
- Greatly important in this respect is GSK3β which is the main target of lithium and several other psychotropic medications.
- Circadian clocks are found throughout the brain and the body and all vital physiological functions are regulated in a rhythmic pattern.
- The prevailing hypothesis posits that disturbances in monoamine transmission, HPA axis function, immunological balance and neurogenesis lead to the development of mood disorders.
- All of these processes are under the control of circadian genes and it is very likely that mood disorders are precipitated in susceptible individuals carrying polymorphisms in these genes.
- By identifying the mechanisms through which components of the circadian system interact with vital physiological processes, it is possible to unravel the neurobiology of psychiatric disorders in general and mood disorders in particular.
- This endeavor would also lead to the discovery of new therapeutic targets for the treatment of chronic psychiatric ailments.

References

1) Kanady JC, Soehnera AM, Harvey AG. A retrospective examination of sleep disturbance across the course of bipolar disorder. J Sleep Disord Ther 2015;4:1000193.
2) Schnell A, Albrecht U, Sandrelli F. Rhythm and mood: relationships between the circadian clock and mood-related behavior. Behav Neurosci 2014;128:326–343.
3) Rumble ME, White KH, Benca RM. Sleep disturbances in mood disorders. Psychiatr Clin North Am. 2015;38:743–759.
4) Levenson JC, Wallace ML, Anderson BP, Kupfer DJ, Frank E. Social rhythm disrupting events increase the risk of recurrence among individuals with bipolar disorder. Bipolar Disord 2015; 17:869–879.
5) Landgraf D, McCarthy MJ, Welsh DK.The role of the circadian clock in animal models of mood disorders. Behav Neurosci 2014; 128:344–359.
6) Borniger JC, Maurya SK, Periasamy M, Nelson RJ. Acute dim light at night increases body mass, alters metabolism, and shifts core body temperature circadian rhythms. Chronobiol Int. 2014;31:917–925.

7) Takahashi JS. Transcriptional architecture of the mammalian circadian clock. Nat Rev Genet 2017;18:164–179.

8) Partch CL, Green CB, Takahashi JS. Molecular architecture of the mammalian circadian clock. Trends Cell Biol 2014;24:90–99.

9) Abreu T, Bragança M. The bipolarity of light and dark: a review on bipolar disorder and circadian cycles. J Affect Disord. 2015;185:219–229.

10) McCarthy MJ, Nievergelt CM, Kelsoe JR, Welsh DK. A survey of genomic studies supports association of circadian clock genes with bipolar disorder spectrum illnesses and lithium response. PLoS One 2012;7:e32091.

11) Abe-Higuchi N, Uchida S, Yamagata H, Higuchi F, Hobara T, Hara K, et al. Hippocampal sirtuin 1 signaling mediates depression-like behavior. Biol Psychiatry 2016;80:815–826.

12) Spencer S, Falcon E, Kumar J, Krishnan V, Mukherjee S, Birnbaum SG, et al. Circadian genes Period 1 and Period 2 in the nucleus accumbens regulate anxiety-related behavior. Eur J Neurosci 2013;37:242–250.

13) Hamon M, Blier P. Monoamine neurocircuitry in depression and strategies for new treatments. Prog Neuropsychopharmacol Biol Psychiatry 2013;45:54–63.

14) Pringle A, Bogdanovskaya M, Waskett P, Zacharia S, Cowen PJ, Harmer CJ. Does melatonin treatment change emotional processing? Implications for understanding the antidepressant mechanism of agomelatine. J Psychopharmacol. 2015;29:1129–1132.

15) Muneer A. Mixed states in bipolar disorder: etiology, pathogenesis and treatment. Chonnam Med J. 2017;53:1–13.

16) Hampp G, Albrecht U. The circadian clock and mood-related behavior. Commun Integr Biol. 2008;1:1–3.

17) Logan RW, Edgar N, Gillman AG, Hoffman D, Zhu X, McClung CA. Chronic stress induces brain region-specific alterations of molecular rhythms that correlate with depression-like behavior in mice. Biol Psychiatry 2015;78:249–258.

18) Kumar S, Chen D, Sehgal A. Dopamine acts through cryptochrome to promote acute arousal in Drosophila. Genes Dev 2012;26:1224–1234.

19) Moon JH, Cho CH, Son GH, Geum D, Chung S, Kim H, et al. Advanced circadian phase in mania and delayed circadian phase in mixed mania and depression returned to normal after treatment of bipolar disorder. EBioMedicine 2016;11:285–295.

20) Al-Hakeim HK, Al-Rammahi DA, Al-Dujaili AH. IL-6, IL-18, sIL-2R, and TNFα proinflammatory markers in depression and schizophrenia patients who are free of overt inflammation. J Affect Disord 2015;182:106–114.

21) Hill AS, Sahay A, Hen R. Increasing adult hippocampal neurogenesis is sufficient to reduce anxiety and depression-like behaviors. Neuropsychopharmacology 2015;40:2368–2378.

22) Mahar I, Bambico FR, Mechawar N, Nobrega JN. Stress, serotonin, and hippocampal neurogenesis in relation to depression and antidepressant effects. Neurosci Biobehav Rev 2014;38:173–192.

23) Curtis AM, Bellet MM, Sassone-Corsi P, O'Neill LA. Circadian clock proteins and immunity. Immunity 2014;40:178–186.

24) Monje FJ, Cabatic M, Divisch I, Kim EJ, Herkner KR, Binder BR, et al. Constant darkness induces IL-6-dependent depression-like behavior through the NF-κB signaling pathway. J Neurosci. 2011;31:9075–9083.

25) Cermakian N, Lange T, Golombek D, Sarkar D, Nakao A, Shibata S, et al. Crosstalk between the circadian clock circuitry and the immune system. Chronobiol Int 2013;30:870–888.

26) McClung CA. Circadian rhythms and mood regulation: insights from pre-clinical models. Eur Neuropsychopharmacol 2011;21 Suppl 4:S683–693.

27) Han DH, Lee YJ, Kim K, Kim CJ, Cho S. Modulation of glucocorticoid receptor induction properties by core circadian clock proteins. Mol Cell Endocrinol 2014;383:170–180.

28) Karlović D, Serretti A, Vrkić N, Martinac M, Marčinko D. Serum concentrations of CRP, IL-6, TNF-α and cortisol in major depressive disorder with melancholic or atypical features. Psychiatry Res 2012;198:74–80.

29) Wiley JW, Higgins GA, Athey BD. Stress and glucocorticoid receptor transcriptional programming in time and space: implications for the brain-gut axis. Neurogastroenterol Motil 2016;28:12–25.

30) Bailey SM, Udoh US, Young ME. Circadian regulation of metabolism. J Endocrinol 2014;222:R75–96.

31) Zwanzger P, Domschke K, Bradwejn J. Neuronal network of panic disorder: the role of the neuropeptide cholecystokinin. Depress Anxiety 2012;29:762–774.

32) Turek FW, Joshu C, Kohsaka A, Lin E, Ivanova G, McDearmon E, et al. Obesity and metabolic syndrome in circadian clock mutant mice. Science 2005;308:1043–1045.

33) Spencer SJ, Xu L, Clarke MA, Lemus M, Reichenbach A, Geenen B, et al. Ghrelin regulates the hypothalamic-pituitary-adrenal axis and restricts anxiety after acute stress. Biol Psychiatry 2012;72:457–65.

34) Kumar J, Chuang JC, Na ES, Kuperman A, Gillman AG, Mukherjee S, et al. Differential effects of chronic social stress and fluoxetine on meal patterns in mice. Appetite 2013;64:81–88.

35) Becker C, Zeau B, Rivat C, Blugeot A, Hamon M, Benoliel JJ. Repeated social defeat-induced depression-like behavioral and biological alterations in rats: involvement of cholecystokinin. Mol Psychiatry 2008;13:1079–92.

36) Arey RN, Enwright JF 3rd, Spencer SM, Falcon E, Ozburn AR, Ghose S, et al. An important role for cholecystokinin, a CLOCK target gene, in the development and treatment of manic-like behaviors. Mol Psychiatry 2014;19:342–50.

37) Barandas R, Landgraf D, McCarthy MJ, Welsh DK. Circadian clocks as modulators of metabolic comorbidity in psychiatric disorders. Curr Psychiatry Rep 2015;17:98.

38) Morris G, Berk M. The many roads to mitochondrial dysfunction in neuroimmune and neuropsychiatric disorders. BMC Med 2015;13:68.

39) Aguilar-Arnal L, Katada S, Orozco-Solis R, Sassone-Corsi P. NAD(+)-SIRT1 control of H3K4 trimethylation through circadian deacetylation of MLL1. Nat Struct Mol Biol 2015 Apr;22:312–318.

40) Um JH, Yang S, Yamazaki S, Kang H, Viollet B, Foretz M, et al. Activation of 5'-AMP-activated kinase with diabetes drug metformin induces casein kinase 1 epsilon (CK1 epsilon)-dependent degradation of clock protein mPer2. J Biol Chem 2007;282:20794–20798.

41) Scarpulla RC. Metabolic control of mitochondrial biogenesis through the PGC-1 family regulatory network. Biochim Biophys Acta 2011;1813:1269–1278.

42) Muneer A. Wnt and GSK3 signaling pathways in bipolar disorder: clinical and therapeutic implications. Clin Psychopharmacol Neurosci 2017;15:100–114.

43) Cole AR. Glycogen synthase kinase 3 substrates in mood disorders and schizophrenia. FEBS J 2013;280:5213–27.

44) Borgs L, Beukelaers P, Vandenbosch R, Nguyen L, Moonen G, Maquet P, et al. Period 2 regulates neural stem/progenitor cell proliferation in the adult hippocampus. BMC Neurosci 2009;10:30.

45) Kott J, Leach G, Yan L. Direction-dependent effects of chronic "jet-lag" on hippocampal neurogenesis. Neurosci Lett 2012;515:177–80.

46) Gilhooley MJ, Pinnock SB, Herbert J. Rhythmic expression of per1 in the dentate gyrus is suppressed by corticosterone: implications for neurogenesis. Neurosci Lett 2011;489(3):177–81.

47) Amare AT, Schubert KO, Klingler-Hoffmann M, Cohen-Woods S, Baune BT. The genetic overlap between mood disorders and cardiometabolic diseases: a systematic review of genome wide and candidate gene studies. Transl Psychiatry 2017;7:e1007.

6 Pathogenesis of Mood Disorders
The Neuroinflammatory Hypothesis

Introduction

Among psychiatric diseases, mood disorders are exclusive in presentation as these patients vacillate between two opposite mood states; that is, mania and depression. More than 70 years ago John Cade serendipitously discovered that lithium had beneficial effects in patients experiencing "mania, dementia praecox and melancholia". The favorable outcome with lithium treatment in patients with major mental illnesses was a breakthrough in that era. Neuroscience has come a long way since that discovery, and research on clinical and preclinical samples have opened new vistas of management for otherwise recalcitrant neuropsychiatric conditions.[1] A cursory appraisal of the currently available psychopharmacological agents would inform us that these medications are based on the monoamine hypothesis of psychiatric disorders. While, undoubtedly, modern drugs provide symptomatic relief and control of acute disease manifestations in a substantial number of patients, these agents fall short of delivering complete cures.[2] Additionally, the available medications carry an enormous burden of adverse effects, tolerability issues and compliance problems. In this scenario the treatment of mental disorders is unsatisfactory, causing huge difficulties for people afflicted by these conditions and placing massive economic burden on society.[3]

Mood disorders are multifaceted medical conditions whose etiology involves genetic and epigenetic factors which act alongside environmental stresses in causing expression of the disease. These diatheses are presently considered as multisystem ailments which affect not only brain functioning but also result in physical comorbidities like cardiovascular disease, diabetes mellitus, disorders of immunity and endocrine dysfunction.[4] Genetic studies have failed to detect any single gene to account for the development of major mood disorders, fostering the prevailing assumption that these are polygenic conditions. Life stresses interact with the involved genes, resulting in epigenetic alterations represented by DNA methylation and chromatin remodeling. These and other modifications imprinting on crucial genes cause disruption in biological and homeostatic mechanisms, resulting in the phenotypic expression of mental disorders.[5] Research efforts in recent years have disclosed that dysregulation of vital biochemical pathways act in an orchestrated manner in the pathogenesis of mood disorders. There is disruption of glucocorticoid signaling, immune-inflammatory imbalance, increased oxidative stress, abnormalities of tryptophan metabolism and derangement of phospholipid turnover with shifts in 1-carbon cycle of methionine and homocysteine. These identified mechanistic pathways offer opportunities for the development of novel and state-of-the-art therapeutic agents, which hold the promise of opening fresh avenues in the treatment of psychiatric disorders in general and mood disorders in particular.[6]

Life stresses acting on predisposed individuals have an enduring effect on the neural substrate causing rewiring of the nervous system with increased sensitization and proneness to recurrent affective episodes. There is growing evidence that manic and major depressive exacerbations have a neurotoxic effect, damaging the neurons as well as the glial elements in the brain. Preclinical and human studies consistently show there is accumulating organ damage both in the center and periphery with illness advancement. The neuroprogressive nature of mood disorders is clinically manifested as increased frequency and severity of episodes, greater suicidal tendency, and cognitive and functional impairments. In the final stages of these diseases there is no illness remission, persistence of inter-episode symptoms and a continued disease state with eventual loss of autonomy.[8] To explain the malignant course of mood disorders, the neuroinflammatory hypothesis has been advanced and it is proposed that the brain is not immune from inflammatory mediators which gain access to this organ and initiate a cascade of pathological changes. The ensuing disturbances include cytokine-induced damage to the neurons, activation of the neurotoxic arm of the kynurenine pathway, increased oxidative stress and generation of free radicals which damage lipids, proteins and nucleic acids. Such toxic events lead to the apoptosis of neurons, decreased density of dendrites and loss of synapses in key mood regulating areas of the brain.[9] It is, therefore mandatory to explore these pathogenic mechanisms, and in the current chapter an earnest effort is made to highlight the most recent finding in this regard. It is surmised that a chronic, low-grade inflammatory process causes disruption in the working of neurons and is responsible for the phenotypic expression of affective illnesses. Figure 6.1 provides an illustrative rendition of the neuroinflammatory hypothesis of mood disorders and shows the progression of events that result in permanent brain damage.

Cytokines and Neuroinflammation

Immune-To-Brain Signaling

During acute affective episodes, patients have elevated levels of inflammatory proteins, i.e., cytokines and chemokines, in the peripheral circulation and this abnormality is well documented in both major depressive disorder (MDD) and bipolar disorder (BD). In this regard, the best studied cytokine

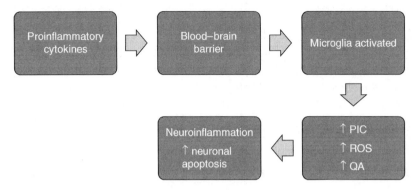

Figure 6.1 The neuroinflammatory hypothesis of mood disorders

The brain is no longer considered immune from peripheral inflammatory processes, since proinflammatory cytokines like IL-6, IL-1β and TNF-α gain access by crossing the blood–brain barrier (BBB). Proinflammatory cytokines activate the microglia which are the primary innate immune cells of the brain. Activated microglia secrete increasing amounts of cytokines, chemokines and reactive oxygen species (ROS) which contribute to further damage by diverting tryptophan metabolism towards production of quinolinic acid (QA) and other neurotoxic kynurenine pathway metabolites. The resulting neuroinflammation leads to apoptosis of neurons, decreased dendritic density and loss of synapses in critical mood regulating areas of the limbic and paralimbic regions. This process is clinically manifested as recognized mood disorder phenotypes.

mediators include interleukin-1 beta (IL-1β), IL-6 and tumor necrosis factor-alpha (TNF-α).[10] These and other inflammatory proteins are liable to incite neuroinflammatory changes through well-described humoral and neural pathways of immune-to-brain signaling. For instance, the humoral pathway may involve blood-borne proinflammatory cytokines provoking inflammation through active transport across the blood–brain barrier, entry into the brain at the circumventricular organ, or binding of cognate receptors on brain endothelial cells with transduction of cytokine signaling into the central nervous system (CNS). In addition, cytokines as well as pathogen-associated molecular patterns (e.g., lipopolysaccharide [LPS]) are capable of stimulating afferent vagal fibers in the periphery, which cause activation of neural pathways in brain regions involved in motivation and mood regulation.[11] Once a peripheral inflammatory signal reaches the brain, microglia, the chief innate immune cells of the CNS, play a pivotal role in mediating the neuroinflammatory response.

Activation of Microglia

The activated microglia intensify the inflammatory response by releasing reactive oxygen species, reactive nitrogen species, cytokines and chemokines. This chemical milieu of oxidative stress and inflammatory signals precipitates a change in astroglial function. Glial indoleamine 2, 3-dioxygenase (IDO), a tryptophan metabolizing enzyme, is upregulated, resulting in greater production of neurotoxic kynurenine metabolites and quinolinic acid (QA) as opposed to 5-HT synthesis.[12] In addition, altered astroglia diminish their neurotrophic production including brain-derived neurotrophic factor (BDNF) and glial cell line-derived neurotrophic factor, and start extruding cytokines and glutamate. Glutamate released from the astroglia accesses extra-synaptic N-methyl D-aspartate (NMDA) receptors, causing suppression of BDNF synthesis and activation of the pro-apoptotic cascade. QA is a potent NMDA agonist that may further potentiate excitotoxicity.[13]

TNF-α Mediated Neurotoxicity

At supra-physiological levels proinflammatory cytokines can directly injure neurons. TNF-α, for instance, interacts with two neuronal receptors, p55 (TNF-RI) and p75 (TNF-RII), and ligand binding to either receptor can activate an apoptotic signaling cascade. The TNF-R then links with the TNF receptor-associated death domain resulting in the recruitment and internalization of Fas, activation of caspase-8, and cell death.[14]

IL-6 Trans-Signaling

IL-6 is a ubiquitous inflammatory cytokine performing diverse biological actions that vary from regeneration and repair of cellular elements to augmenting the response to injury in various types of tissue damage. Several studies have documented an increase in peripheral circulating levels of IL-6 during both acute manic and depressive episodes. IL-6 gains access to the brain from the circulation and stimulates microglia which also secrete this cytokine locally. However, the receptor IL-6R, which it binds to in nanomolar concentrations, is expressed by a few cell types only (including some leukocytes and hepatocytes). The complex of IL-6 and IL-6R combines with a second glycoprotein, gp130 that subsequently dimerizes and kicks off intracellular signaling via the Janus kinase pathway. Unlike IL-6R, gp130 is expressed on all cells; however, the latter alone has no affinity for the cytokine and cells lacking IL-6R cannot respond to this mediator. Of note, a soluble form of IL-6R (sIL-6R) consisting of the extracellular portion of the receptor has been detected in human plasma and other body fluids. sIL-6R is generated by partial proteolysis of the membrane-bound receptor by "a disintegrin and metalloprotease" (ADAM17). The sIL-6R interacts with IL-6 with similar binding properties as the membrane-bound IL-6R. "IL-6 trans-signaling" is the path by which gp130-expressing cells, even in the absence of membrane-bound IL-6R, can be stimulated by the complex of IL-6 and sIL-6R. Because of this phenomenon, the inflammatory process can affect every organ system in the body, including the brain.[15]

Furthermore, experimental models in mice have determined that classic IL-6 signaling has a regenerative and anti-apoptotic role during inflammation, for example in the cecal puncture and ligation sepsis paradigm during which the animals are subjected to extreme stress. In contrast, IL-6 trans-signaling reflects the proinflammatory arm of the cytokine's biological activities. Since the proteolysis of IL-6R is mainly governed by ADAM17, it is highly likely that ADAM17 has a key function in inflammation-related phenomena.

There are important therapeutic implications in this pattern, as specific agents can be developed that block the proinflammatory properties of IL-6 without stalling its anti-inflammatory actions. Many, if not all, neural cells are the target of IL-6 trans-signaling, and inhibition of this activity can be expected to have important beneficial effects in neuropsychiatric disorders. A soluble fusion glycoprotein, sgp130Fc, has been engineered from the extracellular portion of gp130 that exclusively restrains IL-6 trans-signaling. Administration of this engineered protein is a viable treatment approach in major psychiatric conditions, including mood disorders.[16]

The Notion of Sterile Inflammation

It is now known that repeated and severe stressors, in the absence of pathogenic disease, can induce an inflammatory response and this has been aptly called "sterile inflammation". Research in the last decade or so has made it clear that psychological stress, in the non-existence of overt tissue damage, can trigger systemic and CNS sterile inflammation that can have profound damaging effects. This has been substantiated in laboratory animals with such experimental paradigms as social conflict, threat, isolation and rejection which cause increase in C-reactive protein (CRP), proinflammatory cytokines (IL-6, IL-1β, TNF-α) and elevated expression of nuclear factor-κB (NF-κB).[17] The consequence of this proinflammatory state is the expression of depression-like behaviors.

In human subjects parallel findings have been described, for example a study reported that the death of a spouse increased IL-1β and IL-6 activity in older adults with a clinically depressed state.[18] Furthermore, increases in inflammatory markers following exposure to an acute traumatic event is linked to the development, severity and duration of psychiatric disturbances like depression, anxiety and posttraumatic stress disorder.[19] It can be assumed that severe and persistent stress can by itself induce a low-grade inflammatory state, which can precipitate mood perturbation reminiscent of major depression. The inflammatory receptor-ligand interaction invoked in this process is presumed to be between danger associated molecular patterns (DAMP) and inflammasomes, and the ensuing proinflammatory signaling appears to play an overarching role in the pathogenesis of mood disorders.[20]

Inflammatory Molecular Patterns

The main effectors of the inflammatory response are the innate immune cells, while adaptive immune cells are important partners. The former are found throughout the body and CNS and respond to pathogenic organisms, cellular stress and tissue damage. Receptor-ligand recognition schema is a notable and fundamental differentiating attribute between innate and adaptive immune cells. The former use germ-line coded receptors intended to identify conserved molecular patterns and have been named pattern recognition receptors (PRR). A huge number of ligands are capable of binding PRR and include both pathogenic and commensal microbes, termed microbe-associated molecular patterns or MAMP, whereas typically pathogenic patterns are labeled pathogen-associated molecular patterns or PAMP. Examples of MAMP and PAMP include LPS, a membrane incorporated component of many gram negative pathogenic bacteria or CpG DNA, a common viral motif. Of note, a strong inflammatory reaction is the result of PRR-PAMP binding. In contrast to these prototypes, DAMP are endogenous molecules which are increased after cellular stress and tissue damage and PRR-DAMP binding leads to sterile inflammation. Newly recognized DAMP are increasingly being reported and include extracellular heat shock proteins (Hsp), adenosine triphosphate (ATP) and high mobility group box 1 (HMGB1). There is extensive overlap in a broad array of inflammatory proteins that are induced after either LPS (PAMP) or stressor exposure (DAMP). These are detectable in the blood and peripheral tissues and include cytokines, chemokines and mRNA transcripts. In this vein, it should be recognized that brain tissue and microglia also respond to PAMP and DAMP by increasing the secretion of inflammatory mediators.[21]

Sterile Inflammation and the Inflammasome

There is accumulating evidence that acute and intense psychological stress in the absence of obvious tissue damage can provoke a demonstrable local and systemic sterile inflammatory response, with DAMP playing an inciting role. In this respect, tail shock in rodents increases tissue and blood concentration of many cytokines and chemokines, and both MAMP (derived from the gut bacteria) and DAMP signals are involved in the inflammatory response.[22] Significantly, in the said experiments this was attributed to the inflammasome, more specifically the NLRP3 inflammasome known as nucleotide-binding oligomerization domain, leucine rich repeat and pyrin domain protein 3.[23] Inflammasomes are intracellular multi-protein complexes that act as sensors of DAMP and PAMP, causing activation of catalytic caspases and the cleavage and release of proinflammatory cytokines.

For cytokines that are inflammasome independent, the process begins with NF-κB activation after MAMP or DAMP binding to toll-like receptor-4 (TLR-4), CD14 and other potential PRRs. The subsequent signaling cascade comprises of inflammatory gene transcription, translation, protein synthesis and release. In contradistinction, inflammasome dependent cytokine synthesis and release is a two-step process that is initiated after ligation of TLRs and other PRRs leading to NLRP3 gene transcription, translation and protein production. Once the innate immune cells (e.g., microglia) are primed in this way, a second activation signal is required for mature caspase-1 to cleave pro-IL-1β into functional IL-1β, the primary inflammatory mediator of this crucial pathway.[24] The NLRP3 inflammasome appears to react to a wide array of signals (ATP, K+ efflux, β-amyloid, reactive oxygen species, etc.) to get activated and binds to these stimuli as it expresses several PRR including TLR, RAGE (receptor for advanced glycation end products) and CD91. As such it has been incriminated in an extensive range of sterile inflammatory diseases including ischemia-reperfusion injury, autoimmune disorders, diabetes mellitus type II, obesity, atherosclerosis and Alzheimer's disease, conditions which have high comorbidity rates with mood disorders.[25] More specifically, patients with depression had increased expression of NLRP3 and caspase-1 in peripheral blood mononuclear cells, suggesting that sterile inflammation provoked by psychological stress is implicated in the pathogenesis of MDD and other psychopathologies.[26]

Neuroinflammation and Mood Disorders

Microglia perform several crucial functions in the brain including immune-surveillance for pathogens, cellular debris, apoptotic cells and neuronal phenotypic alterations. Upon activation microglia enter a primed position, and when stimulated in this state secrete increased amounts of inflammatory mediators, including IL-1β. As these specialized macrophages express pattern recognition receptors including TLR2 and TLR4, TLR ligation by DAMP (ATP, Hsp, HMGB1, etc.) strongly trigger microglia. Furthermore, several inflammasomes have been described in the microglia including NLRP1, NLRP3 and NLRC4. The NLRP3 inflammasome has been most often studied in the CNS, and is also the focus of the preponderance of studies in animal models of depression. Recent investigations also suggest that NLRP3 may be exquisitely sensitive to the homeostatic perturbations induced by psychobiological stress, with a mechanistic role for the inflammasome mediated processing and maturation of IL-1β in the generation of mood disorders.[27] While space limitation does not allow a detailed description of animal studies highlighting the link between stress, DAMP and the NLRP3 inflammasome, it is clear that CNS inflammation caused by acute or chronic stress has an important role in the development of mood disorders.

Inflammation, Kynurenines and Mood Disorders

The Immune Basis of Mood Disorders

There is limited knowledge regarding the pathophysiology of mood disorders and this is a major obstacle in the discovery of effective preventive and curative therapies. Several converging sources of evidence point to a role for inflammation in the neurobiology of MDD and BD with involvement of a number of biologic systems in the initiation and progression of these conditions. With regards to BD the circulating levels of proinflammatory cytokines have been demonstrated to be increased during the course of acute episodes, returning to baseline with successful mood stabilizing treatment. The strongest support for the contributory role of inflammation in the causation of MDD comes from the observation that cytokine immunotherapy based on chronic administration of interferon-alpha in the treatment of hepatitis C and IL-2 to patients with kidney cancer or melanoma with metastasis, induces an episode of depression in a significant proportion of patients. Further, in the management of resistant mood disorders anti-TNFα treatment with etanercept and infliximab is being explored as an adjunct to standard antidepressants with promising results.[28]

Inflammation and the Kynurenine Pathway

Proinflammatory cytokines activate IDO which is a ubiquitous enzyme that metabolizes tryptophan along the kynurenine pathway. Tryptophan is an essential amino acid obtained from dietary sources; serotonin is synthesized from about 1% of the available tryptophan in the body while the remainder 99% is metabolized in the liver by tryptophan 2, 3 dioxygenase (TDO). TDO action is mainly controlled by the tryptophan level itself and therefore its activity is generally stable and not influenced by inflammatory mediators. During conditions of inflammation and increased oxidative stress, IDO activation in the extra-hepatic tissues shifts the metabolism of tryptophan away from the liver. Kynurenine formed by the action of IDO is further metabolized to compounds which have neuroactive properties. Figure 6.2 shows the main enzymes and products in the kynurenine pathway downstream of IDO.

In circumstances of stress extra kynurenine is formed in the brain *in situ*, whereas its central availability is further enhanced as it can cross the

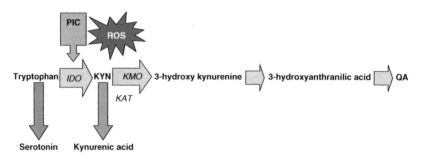

Figure 6.2 The kynurenine pathway of tryptophan metabolism

Tryptophan is the biochemical precursor for the production of serotonin. Activation of the enzyme indoleamine 2, 3 dioxygenase (IDO) by proinflammatory cytokines and reactive oxidative species (ROS) metabolizes tryptophan into kynurenine which can then be metabolized by kynurenine aminotransferase (KAT) into the neuroprotective kynurenic acid or by kynurenine mono-oxygenase (KMO) into the potentially neurotoxic 3-hydroxykynurenine and subsequently to quinolinic acid (QA).

blood–brain barrier. It is worth mentioning that while tryptophan and kynurenine can cross the blood–brain barrier, the rest of the kynurenine metabolites are exclusively formed in the brain itself as these cannot cross from the periphery into the CNS. In summary, under the influence of biological stimuli triggered by stress the kynurenine pathway is highly activated in the brain.[29]

Kynurenines and the Development Of Mood Disorders

Based on the facts presented above, inflammation-induced mood disorders should be amenable to treatment by:

a) Targeting the development of inflammation, for example with cytokine inhibitors or cytokine signaling pathway antagonists.
b) Preventing the formation of peripheral kynurenine with IDO competitive blocker, e.g., 1-methyl tryptophan. In the normal brain up to 78% of kynurenine derives from the blood, while during systemic inflammation nearly all of the brain kynurenine originates from the periphery.
c) Stopping the transport of kynurenine competitively into the brain by increasing the availability of large, branched-chain amino acids.

This approach would certainly work at its best when deployed in a preemptive manner before mood disorders occur. Once an affective episode has come about the neuroactive kynurenine pathway metabolites are formed *in situ* in the brain and an alternate strategy aiming at repairing the inflamed brain has to be put in place.

Neuroactive Properties of the Kynurenine Pathway Metabolites

Among the products of the kynurenine pathway, kynurenic acid has a putative neuroprotective role by acting as an antagonist of NMDA receptors, while it also decreases glutamate levels via inhibition of α7 nicotinic receptors. 3-hydroxykynurenine is a free radical generator, and QA is an NMDA receptor agonist that also exerts neurotoxic effects via lipid peroxidation and disruption of the blood–brain barrier. The neurotoxic activity of QA has been known for more than 30 years and this metabolite should *a priori* be a therapeutic target by blocking its formation or antagonizing its excitotoxic effect on NMDA glutamatergic receptors. However, in the context of an inflamed brain the microglia are activated which release large quantities of glutamate, a process facilitated by the uptake of extracellular glutamine that is converted to glutamate by the enzyme glutaminase. Moreover, oxidative stress generated by 3-hydroxykynurenine and 3-hydroxyanthranilic acid further contributes to microglia priming. In the normal brain the clearance of glutamate is efficient as astrocytes uptake this substance and convert it to glutamine via glutamine synthetase which is recycled back to neurons for the continued formation of glutamate. However, in conditions of excitotoxicity the extracellular concentration of glutamate can increase up to 100 fold, overwhelming this mechanism of glutamate reprocessing. Such pathologically increased levels of glutamate result in atrophic changes in key mood regulating areas like the hippocampus and amygdala.[30]

Promising Strategies for Treating Mood Disorders

An important mechanism for the clearance of brain extracellular glutamate is represented by the efflux of glutamate from the brain interstitial fluid into the blood. The brain-to-blood efflux of glutamate is limited by the relatively high levels of plasma glutamate, so that an efficient way to substantially enhance this process is to accelerate the degradation of glutamate in the blood by administering oxaloacetate that activates glutamic oxaloacetate transaminase (GOT). This enzyme catalyzes the transformation of glutamate into 2-ketoglutarate. Blood glutamate scavenging can be enhanced further by adding recombinant GOT to oxaloacetate. The neuroprotective effect of blood glutamate scavenging has been confirmed in a number of experimental conditions associated with high brain concentrations of glutamate, such as traumatic brain injury, epilepsy and ischemic stroke.[31]

Finally, to achieve personalized treatments for mood disorders, it is necessary to develop suitable biomarkers for identifying patients who are the most likely to benefit from targeting the sequence of events leading from inflammation to MDD and BD. The events to be marked in this chain are the transport of kynurenine into the brain, the production and action of kynurenine metabolites particularly QA, and possibly the increased concentrations of glutamate in the brain interstitial fluids.

Purported Model of Depression

A proposed model of depression is presented as follows:[32]

1) Exposure to stressors results in the release of DAMP within the brain, presumably from damaged or dying neurons.
2) These neuron-derived DAMP then target their cognate receptors on microglia leading to NLRP3 inflammasome activation and the synthesis and release of inflammatory mediators, including IL-1β.
3) The secreted form of this cytokine may drive the induction of IDO.
4) IDO-mediated catabolism of tryptophan feeds into the kynurenine pathway, thereby diverting the pool of this essential amino acid from 5-HT synthesis to potentially neurotoxic metabolites and reducing the availability of the neurotransmitter.
5) Decreased availability of serotonin provokes a depressive phenotype with attendant psychological, neuro-vegetative and somatic symptoms.

As a summarizing note, it must be appreciated that understanding the processes involving sterile inflammation, DAMP/MAMP/PAMP signaling in the periphery and CNS and inflammasome activation are critical for efficacious therapeutics of affective disorders. While notable advances are made in this respect in neurological disorders such as stroke, novel agents have not yet been tested in psychiatric patients. New therapeutic modalities emerging from enhanced knowledge can pave the way for curative treatments for otherwise intractable conditions. Figure 6.3 gives a schematic representation of this supposed model of depression and depicts the key role of NLRP3 inflammasome and IL-1β in the expression of the depressive phenotype.

Oxidative Stress

Physiological Role of Free Radicals

Oxidative stress is defined as a persistent imbalance between antioxidants and pro-oxidants in favor of the latter. The result of this disparity is the excessive production of free radicals, the reactive oxygen species (ROS). Nevertheless, at low physiological concentrations ROS perform important functions in the CNS. These include regulation of neuronal fate through differentiation and death via the activation of activator protein-1 transcription factor which in turn mediates the nerve growth factor pathways. ROS are involved in crucial signaling cascades such as the control of the membrane potential and cellular H^+ fluxes, the execution of cardiovascular homeostasis and management of blood pressure through the angiotensin II receptor, and the regulation of the glutamatergic neurotransmission via the NMDA receptor. Additionally, ROS are involved in the neuroinflammatory response by means of priming of the microglia. Redox signaling may have a key role in coordinating the responses of the neuronal cells to deal with adverse stimuli, either by promoting resilience through stress-induced molecular cascades such as the mitogen activated protein kinase or by eliminating the seriously damaged cells through apoptosis.[33]

Pathophysiological Mechanisms

On the other hand, the accumulation of ROS is known to increase the susceptibility of brain tissue to damage and purportedly play a central role in the pathophysiology of several neuropsychiatric disorders. Clear evidence of the involvement of increased brain oxidative damage has been reported for neurodegenerative conditions like Alzheimer's and Parkinson's diseases, cerebrovascular disorders, demyelinating diseases and major psychiatric disorders such as schizophrenia, MDD and BD. ROS cause glutamate excitotoxicity and alter mitochondrial activity. Mitochondrial dysfunction in turn causes NMDA receptor upregulation and further increased oxidative stress, finally leading to a detrimental vicious cellular cycle. Oxidative stress products such as superoxide and

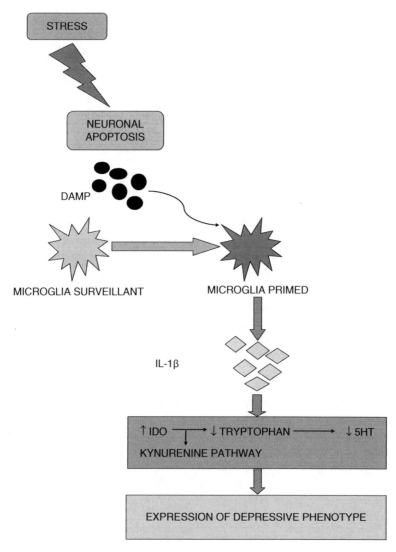

Figure 6.3   Stress-induced sterile inflammation and expression of the depressive phenotype

In a supposed model of depression, psychological stressors cause damage to neurons with efflux of a broad range of signals or damage associated molecular patterns (DAMPs). These bind to pattern recognition receptors such as toll-like receptors (TLR 2/4) and purigenic receptors (P2X7R) on microglia and cause the formation of NLRP3 inflammasomes via transcription, translation and protein synthesis. Primed microglia release mature IL-1β via activated inflammasomes, and furthermore this proinflammatory cytokine induces the enzyme indoleamine 2, 3 dioxygenase (IDO). The latter catabolizes tryptophan, an essential amino acid required in the synthesis of serotonin. Diversion of tryptophan metabolism towards the kynurenine pathway leads to a decrease of serotonin, as well as the formation of potentially neurotoxic metabolites like quinolinic acid (QA). As a final step, reduction of this key neurotransmitter at the synapse leads to the provocation of sickness behavior and depressive symptoms.

hydroxyl radicals have been shown to induce cortisol resistance by impairing the translocation of the glucocorticoid receptor from the cytosol to the nucleus. HPA axis dysregulation by ROS in turn causes a proinflammatory response with increased circulating levels of proinflammatory cytokines. Unrestricted ROS activity is also responsible for increased blood–brain barrier permeability through launching of matrix metalloproteinases and subsequent degradation of tight junctions. This results in increased access of inflammatory mediators to the brain tissue leading to unrepressed neuroinflammation and neuronal death.[34]

Redox Balance in the Brain

The assumed pathophysiological relationship between oxidative stress and mood disorders may be due to the fact that the nervous system is particularly vulnerable to oxidative damage for the following reasons:

1) The brain has the highest consumption rate of oxygen of all the organs; it is roughly 2% of the body weight but uses 20% of the total inspired oxygen. This fact predisposes it to greater production of free radicals during the process of mitochondrial energy metabolism.
2) The brain's lipid content is very high which acts as a substrate for the ROS.
3) There exists the redox potential of several neurotransmitters, for instance dopamine.
4) The defense systems against free radicals are relatively inefficient.
5) The brain has a high content of metal ions, for example iron and copper, involved in redox reactions.

The protective arrangement against pro-oxidants is composed of an enzymatic and a non-enzymatic component. Glutathione peroxidase and glutathione reductase are well-known intracellular antioxidant enzymes. The former converts peroxides and hydroxyl radicals into nontoxic forms, often with the concomitant oxidation of reduced glutathione (GSH) into the oxidized form glutathione disulfide (GSSG), and glutathione reductase recycles GSSG to GSH. Other enzymes and pathways are also involved in the management of cellular resistance against oxidative stress, notably catalase (CAT) and superoxide dismutase (SOD), which acting in concert with glutathione peroxidase constitute the major defense or primary antioxidant enzymes against superoxide radicals. In addition, glutathione-S-transferase and glucose-6-phosphate dehydrogenase are important in maintaining a steady supply of metabolic intermediates like GSH and nicotinamide adenine dinucleotide-phosphate (NADPH) necessary for optimum functioning of the primary antioxidant enzymes.[35]

Measurement of Oxidative Stress

The main ROS include the superoxide radical (O_2-), hydrogen peroxide (H_2O_2) and hydroxyl radical ($OH\cdot$). Interaction between ROS and nitric oxide results in the formation of highly reactive nitrogen species (RNS), such as the peroxynitrite ions (ONOO⁻) which are very damaging to the basic structural molecules of the cells. Because ROS and RNS have extremely short half-lives, these are difficult to quantify. Therefore, it is necessary to search for and determine indirect pointers of oxidative stress; these include lipid, protein and DNA peroxidation indicators, while measurement of key enzymes involved in the neutralization of free radicals also serve as putative markers. Biosignatures of oxidative stress in body fluids include oxidized proteins like protein carbonyls and oxidized lipids such as 4-hydroxynonenol, thiobarbituric acid reactive substances, malondialdehyde and isoprostanes which are isomers resulting from the oxidation of arachidonic acid. Neuroprostanes are also emerging as specific biomarkers of oxidative stress in the CNS. In addition, oxidation of DNA at the guanine residue site produces 8-hydroxydeoxyguanosine which is associated with telomere shortening detectable in peripheral blood cells or fibroblasts. Telomere shortening is an indicator of accelerated aging with increased incidence of comorbid conditions like cardiovascular diseases in major psychiatric conditions, including mood disorders. There is consistent evidence from peripheral marker studies that the brain's primary antioxidants, GSH, CAT, SOD and GSH peroxidase are altered in patients with affective illnesses. Further, there is now meta-analysis level data showing increased pointers of oxidative stress. The most dependable findings are increased lipid peroxidation, nucleic acid damage and raised nitric oxide in mood disorder patients compared to controls, with high effect sizes for lipid peroxidation.[36]

NADPH Oxidase Enzymes as a Potential Therapeutic Target

NADPH oxidase (NOX) enzymes whose sole purpose is the generation of ROS, are emerging as an important source of oxidative stress in major psychiatric disorders. These function in the trans-membrane electron transport chain using cytoplasmic NADPH as an electron donor to molecular O_2, generating ROS in the extracellular space or the lumen of intracellular organelles. Seven NOX genes have been identified, the best described isoform being NOX2. NOX enzymes are widely distributed in a variety of tissues and presence of NOX transcripts have been confirmed in total brain samples as well as in neurons, microglia and astrocytes. In the presence of severe life stress (SLS), these enzymes are induced causing increased production of ROS in the brain and contribute to the expression of the main psychiatric diseases including MDD and BD. Animal experiments in rodents and primates with such paradigms as social isolation and establishment of communal hierarchy models have been very helpful in showing the role of NOX enzymes in causing oxidative damage and leading to different types of abnormal behavior. In the case of long-lasting, chronic SLS the neurophysiologic impact of excessive ROS generation gives rise to persistent excitatory, glutamatergic transmission leading to changes reminiscent of alterations observed in patients with psychotic spectrum conditions. These include NMDA receptor downregulation,

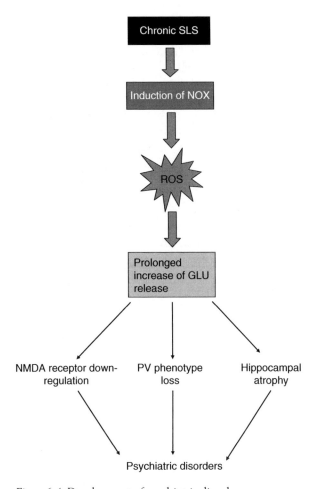

Figure 6.4 Development of psychiatric disorders as a consequence of prolonged SLS

When subjected to long-lasting severe life stress (SLS) pathophysiological changes take place in the brain. NADPH oxidase (NOX) enzymes are induced, particularly NOX2, with ensuing increased generation of reactive oxygen species (ROS). The latter enhance the release of glutamate (GLU) from neurons; prolonged glutamatergic discharge has such resultant effects as N-methyl D-aspartate (NMDA) receptor downregulation, loss of phenotype of inhibitory parvalbumin (PV) interneurons and apoptotic changes in the hippocampus. These alterations are similar to those seen in psychosis; the putative model of major psychiatric disorders described here is extrapolated from animal experiments carried out in rodents and primates.

failure of inhibitory phenotype of GABAergic interneurons, and reduction of hippocampal volume.[37] At least, in some animal models the source of oxidative stress has been shown to be the increased expression of NOX enzymes and if confirmed in humans, it might prove to be a promising target for drug development. Figure 6.4 illustrates this supposed model of disease development.

Conclusion

A large body of evidence incriminates immune-inflammatory mechanisms in the induction and progression of major mood disorders. Several meta-analyses published in the past few years support evidence of raised inflammatory markers during acute affective episodes. However, there is a lingering question: whether heightened inflammation is present in every patient or is this phenomenon limited to a subset of patients with mood disorders? In the light of extant evidence a justified observation would be that inflammatory processes are more evident in patients who show increased severity of affective disturbances, but a chronic, low-grade disturbance continues even in euthymic periods. This line of argument could explain the systemic nature of mood disorders, the increased frequency of these conditions in subjects exposed to childhood maltreatment and the fact that decrease in inflammatory markers is associated with a successful treatment response. The challenge for neuroscience is to unravel the pathogenic processes that lead to the development of major mood disorders. By pinpointing the disease-producing mechanisms, it would be possible to find new cures for these and other neuropsychiatric conditions. While it is true that currently available medications based on the monoamine hypothesis of mood disorders have offered temporary respite to a certain percentage of patients, many patients are treatment refractory. Therefore, there is an urgent need for new agents which are based on fresh perceptions and target biological pathways that play a crucial role in provoking these conditions.

Summary Points

- Clinical and animal studies increasingly incriminate immune-inflammatory imbalance in the development of major mood disorders.
- Greater immune disturbance is associated with increased severity of affective episodes, suicidal tendencies, progressive course and poor health outcomes.
- Efficacious treatment of mood disorders is associated with an accompanying reduction in markers of inflammation.
- The neuroinflammatory hypothesis of mood disorders posits that pro-inflammatory mediators gain access to the brain and trigger microglia, which are the innate immune cells of this organ.
- A cascade of pathogenic changes ensues characterized by deranged tryptophan metabolisms, mitochondrial dysfunction, increased oxidative stress and the production of damaging free radicals.
- The ultimate consequence is apoptosis of neurons, reduction in dendrite density and loss of synapses in crucial mood regulating regions of the brain.
- For better therapeutics, novel agents are needed which target the pathogenic chain of events involved in the development of mood disorders.

References

1) Horsdal HT, Köhler-Forsberg O, Benros ME, Gasse C. C-reactive protein and white blood cell levels in schizophrenia, bipolar disorders and depression – associations with mortality and psychiatric outcomes: a population-based study. Eur Psychiatry 2017;44:164–172.

2) Ashok AH, Marques TR, Jauhar S, Nour MM, Goodwin GM, Young AH, Howes OD. The dopamine hypothesis of bipolar affective disorder: the state of the art and implications for treatment. Mol Psychiatry 2017;22:666–679.

3) Karpov B, Joffe G, Aaltonen K, Suvisaari J, Baryshnikov I, Näätänen P, et al. Level of functioning, perceived work ability, and work status among psychiatric patients with major mental disorders. Eur Psychiatry 2017;44:83–9.

4) Saavedra K, Molina-Márquez AM, Saavedra N, Zambrano T, Salazar LA. Epigenetic modifications of major depressive disorder. Int J Mol Sci 2016;17:E1279.

5) Kim HD, Hesterman J, Call T, Magazu S, Keeley E, Armenta K, et al. SIRT1 mediates depression-like behaviors in the nucleus accumbens. J Neurosci 2016;36:8441–8452.

6) Won E, Kim YK. Stress, the autonomic nervous system, and the immune-kynurenine pathway in the etiology of depression. Curr Neuropharmacol 2016;14:665–673.

7) Walker AJ, Kim Y, Price JB, Kale RP, McGillivray JA, Berk M, et al. Stress, inflammation, and cellular vulnerability during early stages of affective disorders: biomarker strategies and opportunities for prevention and intervention. Front Psychiatry 2014;5:34.

8) Verduijn J, Milaneschi Y, van Hemert AM, Schoevers RA, Hickie IB, Penninx BW, et al. Clinical staging of major depressive disorder: an empirical exploration. J Clin Psychiatry 2015;76:1200–1208.

9) Kaufmann FN, Costa AP, Ghisleni G, Diaz AP, Rodrigues ALS, Peluffo H, et al. NLRP3 inflammasome-driven pathways in depression: clinical and preclinical findings. Brain Behav Immun 2017;64:367–383.

10) Tu PC, Li CT, Lin WC, Chen MH, Su TP, Bai YM. Structural and functional correlates of serum soluble IL-6 receptor level in patients with bipolar disorder. J Affect Disord 2017;219:172–177.

11) Lichtblau N, Schmidt FM, Schumann R, Kirkby KC, Himmerich H. Cytokines as biomarkers in depressive disorder: current standing and prospects. Int Rev Psychiatry 2013;25:592–603.

12) Müller N. Immunological aspects of the treatment of depression and schizophrenia. Dialogues Clin Neurosci 2017;19:55–63.

13) Kim YK, Won E. The influence of stress on neuroinflammation and alterations in brain structure and function in major depressive disorder. Behav Brain Res 2017;329:6–11.

14) Szuster-Ciesielska A, Słotwińska M, Stachura A, Marmurowska-Michałowska H, Dubas-Slemp H, Bojarska-Junak A, et al. Accelerated apoptosis of blood leukocytes and oxidative stress in blood of patients with major depression. Prog Neuropsychopharmacol Biol Psychiatry 2008;32:686–94.

15) Maes M, Anderson G, Kubera M, Berk M. Targeting classical IL-6 signalling or IL-6 trans-signalling in depression? Expert OpinTher Targets. 2014;18:495–512.

16) Fonseka TM, McIntyre RS, Soczynska JK, Kennedy SH. Novel investigational drugs targeting IL-6 signaling for the treatment of depression. Expert Opin Investig Drugs 2015;24:459–475.

17) Su WJ, Zhang Y, Chen Y, Gong H, Lian YJ, Peng W, et al. NLRP3 gene knockout blocks NF-κB and MAPK signaling pathway in CUMS-induced depression mouse model. Behav Brain Res 2017;322:1–8.

18) Schultz-Florey CR, Martinez-Maza O, Magpantay L, Breen EC, Irwin MR, Gundel H, et al. When grief makes you sick: bereavement induced systemic inflammation is a question of genotype. Brain Behav Immun 2012;26:1066–1071.

19) Mills NT, Scott JG, Wray NR, Cohen-Woods S, Baune BT. Research review: the role of cytokines in depression in adolescents: a systematic review. J Child Psychol Psychiatry 2013;54:816–835.

20) Alcocer-Gómez E, Castejón-Vega B, Cordero MD. Stress-induced NLRP3 inflammasome in human diseases. Adv Protein Chem Struct Biol 2017;108:127–162.

21) Abderrazak A, Syrovets T, Couchie D, El Hadri K, Friguet B, Simmet T, et al. NLRP3 inflammasome: from a danger signal sensor to a regulatory node of oxidative stress and inflammatory diseases. Redox Biol 2015;4:296–307.

22) Maslanik T, Mahaffey L, Tannura K, Beninson L, Greenwood BN, Fleshner M. The inflammasome and danger associated molecular patterns (DAMPs) are implicated in cytokine and chemokine responses following stressor exposure. Brain Behav Immun 2013;28:54–62.

23) Fleshner M, Frank M, Maier SF. Danger signals and inflammasomes: stress-evoked sterile inflammation in mood disorders. Neuropsychopharmacology 2017;42:36–45.

24) Pan Y, Chen XY, Zhang QY, Kong LD. Microglial NLRP3 inflammasome activation mediates IL-1β-related inflammation in prefrontal cortex of depressive rats. Brain Behav Immun 2014;41:90–100.

25) Lee HM, Kim JJ, Kim HJ, Shong M, Ku BJ, Jo EK. Upregulated NLRP3 inflammasome activation in patients with type 2 diabetes. Diabetes 2013;62:194–204.

26) Alcocer-Gómez E, de Miguel M, Casas-Barquero N, Núñez-Vasco J, Sánchez-Alcazar JA, Fernández-Rodríguez A, et al. NLRP3 inflammasome is activated in mononuclear blood cells from patients with major depressive disorder. Brain Behav Immun 2014;36:111–117.

27) Weber MD, Frank MG, Tracey KJ, Watkins LR, Maier SF. Stress induces the danger-associated molecular pattern HMGB-1 in the hippocampus of male Sprague Dawley rats: a priming stimulus of microglia and the NLRP3 inflammasome. J Neurosci 2015;35:316–324.

28) Réus GZ, Fries GR, Stertz L, Badawy M, Passos IC, Barichello T, et al. The role of inflammation and microglial activation in the pathophysiology of psychiatric disorders. Neuroscience 2015;300:141–154.

29) Réus GZ, Jansen K, Titus S, Carvalho AF, Gabbay V, Quevedo J. Kynurenine pathway dysfunction in the pathophysiology and treatment of depression: evidences from animal and human studies. J Psychiatr Res 2015;68:316–328.

30) Savitz J. Role of kynurenine metabolism pathway activation in major depressive disorders. Curr Top Behav Neurosci 2017;31:249–267.

31) Dantzer R, Walker AK. Is there a role for glutamate-mediated excitotoxicity in inflammation-induced depression? J Neural Transm (Vienna) 2014;121:925–932.

32) Fleshner M. Stress-evoked sterile inflammation, danger associated molecular patterns (DAMPs), microbial associated molecular patterns (MAMPs) and the inflammasome. Brain Behav Immun 2013;27:1–7.

33) Park J, Min JS, Kim B, Chae UB, Yun JW, Choi MS, et al. Mitochondrial ROS govern the LPS-induced pro-inflammatory response in microglia cells by regulating MAPK and NF-κB pathways. Neurosci Lett. 2015;584:191–196.

34) Hernandes MS, D'Avila JC, Trevelin SC, Reis PA, Kinjo ER, Lopes LR, et al. The role of Nox2-derived ROS in the development of cognitive impairment after sepsis. J Neuroinflammation 2014;11:36.

35) Popa-Wagner A, Mitran S, Sivanesan S, Chang E, Buga AM. ROS and brain diseases: the good, the bad, and the ugly. Oxid Med Cell Longev 2013;2013:963520.

36) Black CN, Bot M, Scheffer PG, Cuijpers P, Penninx BW. Is depression associated with increased oxidative stress? A systematic review and meta-analysis. Psychoneuroendocrinology 2015;51:164–175.

37) Liang D, Li G, Liao X, Yu D, Wu J, Zhang M. Developmental loss of parvalbumin-positive cells in the prefrontal cortex and psychiatric anxiety after intermittent hypoxia exposures in neonatal rats might be mediated by NADPH oxidase-2. Behav Brain Res 2016;296:134–140.

7   Staging and Neuroprogression of Mood Disorders

Introduction

Mood disorders are severe neuropsychiatric ailments characterized by onset in adolescence or early adulthood, recurrent course and a lifelong duration. The patients experience continual vacillations in energy levels, affect, sleep and the psychological state.[1] The diathesis has a pervasive negative effect on all aspects of patients' lives as they experience social, psychological, academic and occupational difficulties because of the underlying mood disturbance. Since these are persistent and progressive conditions, there is an immense need to stage define mood disorders, as it helps in better understanding the disease trajectory, as well as delivering personalized treatments.[2]

There is increasing evidence to demonstrate that major mood disorders are phasic in nature, exemplified by such epochs as a prodrome, a symptomatic period and a residual state. Many authors have underscored the problem of delay in initial identification which is of the magnitude of several years in some cases, due to misdiagnosis and giving of wrong labels to these patients.[3] Inappropriate or inadequate treatment as a result of this reason can result in repeated mood exacerbations, continual subthreshold symptoms, and the development of complications such as substance abuse. This cycle of disease advancement leads to cognitive impairment, functional decline and loss of essential skills required in the performance of daily tasks.[4] There is mounting proof that manic and major depressive episodes have a toxic effect on neurons and glia, producing permanent pathological changes in the regions of brain critical in mood regulation. The neuroprogressive nature of mood disorders can be arrested with early diagnosis, proper treatment on the biopsychosocial lines, recognition of neuropsychiatric and physical comorbidities and individually tailored management according to the phase of the illness.[5] In this respect, it is imperative to demarcate the stages of the disorder to facilitate the delivery of improved patient care and attain better outcomes for patients. It must be emphasized that the staging approach has been highly beneficial in the overall management of other complex (gene × environment) disorders including diabetes, cardiovascular disease and various forms of cancer.

Staging presupposes that illness advances in an identifiable temporal progression of phases from an at-risk, prodromal period to the first clinical manifestations, and further develops into more severe, intractable forms with evolution and chronicity.[6] Current diagnostic systems emphasize presenting symptoms with a categorical and cross-sectional approach without considering the context, the preceding risk factors and neglecting what is known about the natural history of illness development. More than a century ago, Kraepelin first realized that psychiatric disorders had a staged development and his view of their progressive nature was reflected in his nomenclature of dementia praecox and manic depressive insanity. Regarding the latter, he recognized that while the initial episodes were frequently precipitated by stressful events followed by complete improvement, as the illness evolved the patients had affective recurrences in the absence of stressful experiences and did not show full inter-episode recovery.[7]

Clinical staging is a useful conceptual framework to refine the phenotype of illness along developmental lines and supports the identification of trait- and state-specific biomarkers. It paves the way for stratified and personalized treatment at each stage of the illness as is happening in other branches of medicine. With regards to progressive conditions like mood disorders early intervention is likely to be simpler and more effective and aims to significantly prevent or delay advancement to more severe presentations requiring complex treatment strategies which are less acceptable to patients and have a lower benefit-to-risk ratio.[8] In spite of the obvious benefits of clinical staging, this aspect of illness classification has been neglected in psychiatry until recently. However, there is now an increased impetus to characterize by stages major psychiatric disorders, including mood disorders. In this respect, staging models have been proposed by different researchers incorporating the longitudinal history of affective illnesses from a high-risk prodromal period to illness progression to more severe and refractory states. In this chapter an earnest effort is made to bring to light the latest understanding of the staging models of major mood disorders and the related concept of neuroprogression. The clinical and biological findings are described to reconcile the two phenomena and demonstrate the practical advantages of incorporating these notions in everyday practice.

Developmental Trajectory and Clinical Heterogeneity of Mood Disorders

Classical, Recurrent Bipolar Disorder

Bipolar Disorder (BD) is currently viewed as a spectrum illness which includes several phenotypes. The classic BD is typified by recurrent mood episodes of opposite polarity with full inter-episode recovery, very high heritability and a good response to lithium in up to 80% of cases.[9] It is not associated with cognitive and functional decline and is characterized by a relative absence of psychiatric comorbidities like anxiety and substance use disorders. The family history of patients with classical BD is marked by high genetic predisposition in that they usually have a parent or a close relative with a similar condition. As children and adolescents they may show an excess of adjustment, sleep and anxiety disorders such as circadian rhythm sleep disorders and separation anxiety disorder.[10] The offspring of classical, lithium-responsive BD patients are often gifted, have a completely normal early development with good academic and social adjustment. In rare cases classic, lithium-responsive BD may occur in individuals without a family history of the condition but this would be an exception rather than the rule. The frequency of recurrences and the quality of remission are known to vary substantially between patients; however, over time there is no significant change in illness phase and polarity, absence of cycle acceleration and lack of subthreshold affective symptoms between episodes. This phenotype is marked by an absence of evidence for progressive worsening of the course; furthermore, there may be an increased incidence of recurrent mood disorders but not schizophrenia in the relatives. In one sample of outpatients, this comprised of 30% of the total BD patients seen in a subspecialty clinic of a Canadian teaching hospital.[11] The classical episodic lithium-responsive subtype now forms part of a much broader spectrum of BD.

Bipolar Spectrum Disorders

Evidence supports that bipolar subtypes defined by either prophylactic response or nonresponse to lithium differ in clinical course, family history and neurobiological correlates. Lithium nonresponsive subtypes are more chronic disorders that preferentially respond to atypical neuroleptics, merging into psychotic spectrum conditions. Alternatively, some bipolar spectrum patients respond to anticonvulsants as in the case of BD type II with comorbid anxiety disorders.[12] BD with psychotic symptoms has overlapping neurobiological findings with schizophrenia spectrum disorders and a higher risk of having chronic non-affective psychoses in family members. In help-seeking symptomatic youth, the illness trajectory of non-classical BD is marked by negative symptoms like affective flattening, anhedonia, apathy and social withdrawal, overlapping clinically with depressive disorders. They are liable to neurodevelopmental disorders including learning disabilities, attentional problems, academic failure and may exhibit cluster A personality traits.[13] The illness course of these young bipolar patients may be progressive, marked by mixed episodes, incomplete remissions, persistent subthreshold symptoms, cognitive impairments and functional decline in the latter stages of the illness. There is evidence for a continual proinflammatory state, increased level of oxidative stress and failing neurotrophic support.[14] Neuroimaging studies show increased volume of lateral ventricles with loss of brain matter in the final stages of the disease.

Youth Precursors of Bipolar Disorder

BD is not diagnosed until the occurrence of the first manic or hypomanic episode; however, the bipolar diathesis most often starts with a depressive episode which may antecede the first diagnosable activated episode by many years. A positive family history informs the risk of BD in youth who present with melancholic depressive episodes. There are other antecedents which include nonspecific anxiety syndromes, and persistent mood instability diagnosable only as depressive disorder not otherwise specified, cyclothymia or emotional dysregulation.[15] In addition, in samples of help-seeking youth attenuated psychotic symptoms, and attentional and cognitive problems often coexist along with affective symptoms.[16] The early forerunners are nonspecific and are seen in other illness trajectories including psychotic disorders, internalizing and externalizing disorders, and substance use disorders. These can also be self-limited presentations in some young people and may not progress to major psychiatric illnesses. However, it is the nature of the family history that brings important context to the otherwise vague clinical manifestation in children and adolescents.[17] The history of BD in close family members and their response to specific treatments, for example lithium, are important predictive factors aiding in the early differentiation of illness trajectories and in foretelling treatment outcome in symptomatic youth. As a cautionary note, stimulants and antidepressants should be either avoided or, if used, kept to low doses, short duration and closely monitored in young patients with a confirmed family history of BD.[18]

Prospective Studies of Offspring of Parents with Bipolar Disorder

A number of longitudinal, prospective studies of offspring of parents with confirmed diagnosis of BD have shown divergence in illness course based on subtypes of the illness. Specifically, children of BD parents with an excellent response to long-term lithium had a completely normal or endowed early developmental course. In contrast, the children of parents who failed to respond to lithium prophylaxis manifested childhood problems with cognition, emotional regulation, socialization and had neurodevelopmental disorders.[19] Among high-risk offspring who developed major mood disorders, the children of lithium responders had an episodic, remitting course and responded to lithium prophylaxis, while the offspring of lithium nonresponders exhibited a non-remitting course and responded preferentially to either prophylaxis with an anticonvulsant or an atypical antipsychotic. Moreover, the spectrum of end-stage disorders among the affected offspring of lithium responders was limited to mood disorders, while the offspring of lithium nonresponders showed both mood and psychotic spectrum illnesses.[20] The analysis, based on up to 17 years of prospective clinical research observation, holds up that BD develops in a sequence of predictable clinical phases; not all offspring manifest all stages, but once they enter the model they proceed in a forward sequence. The clinical staging model is a collective overview, and it should be kept in mind that not all high-risk offspring follow the same illness trajectory or advance to end-stage illness.[21]

Major Depressive Disorder

In contrast, MDD is a somewhat more homogeneous condition. The age of onset is usually later, in the twenties and early thirties and the patients follow

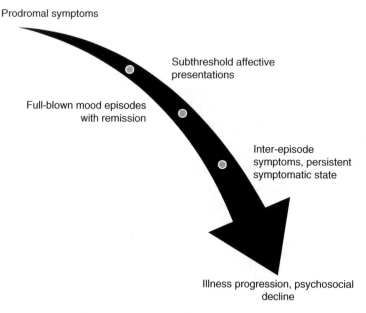

Prodromal symptoms

Subthreshold affective
presentations

Full-blown mood episodes
with remission

Inter-episode
symptoms, persistent
symptomatic state

Illness progression, psychosocial
decline

Figure 7.1 Schema to stage define disease advancement in mood disorders

There are childhood antecedents to mood disorders, exemplified by such disturbances as non-specific anxiety, sleep and adjustment disorders. In about one-third of patients, the course is relatively benign with response to classical mood stabilizers and standard antidepressants. However, the majority of patients with mood disorders have an advancing diathesis which is ultimately manifested as pathological brain changes and severe decline in the biopsychosocial realm of functioning. See text for further details.

a remitting and relapsing course, exhibiting unipolar depressive episodes only. The prevalence of general medical and neuropsychiatric comorbidities is also lower. There is a high rate of conversion to BD type I or BD type II on longitudinal follow-up, and even in patients who continue to have unipolar depressive episodes, many show additional benefit with the adjunctive use of mood stabilizers and atypical antipsychotics along with standard antidepressants. There is definite evidence that severe, recurrent major depressive episodes lead to neuroprogressive changes in the brain, and in this regard atrophy of the hippocampal neurons and decreased neurogenesis in the dentate gyrus are well-replicated findings. In view of the extant evidence it is fair to assume that MDD is also an advancing diathesis amenable to the staging paradigm, with essentially similar connotations for the two major mood disorders.[22] Figure 7.1 is a schematic representation of the basic notion behind staging of mood disorders.

Neuroprogression as the Basis for Staging Mood Disorders

There is ample research evidence that affective illnesses are evolving conditions in which early stages have different clinical features compared to later phases. The advancement of the diathesis, frequently connected with such factors as misdiagnosis and inadequate treatment, is associated with greater frequency of episodes which start occurring spontaneously with disease progression. Recurrent and severe affective episodes are linked to higher rates of comorbidities, increased risk of suicide, more hospitalizations and treatment resistance. Accompanying these phenomena are cognitive deterioration and functional decline in such areas as occupation, social relationships and financial independence with eventual loss of autonomy.[23] Research efforts in the last few decades have begun to unravel the neurobiological correlates of the worsening clinical course in mood disorders. The term "neuroprogression" has been increasingly used to define the pathological reorganization of the central nervous system which results from various insults, such as inflammation and oxidative stress. In mood disorders neural substrate reactivity is changed by repeated mood episodes, ultimately promoting a brain rewiring that leads to an increased vulnerability to life stresses. An episode-dependent deterioration pattern has been widely described in serum biomarkers, brain imaging and neuropsychological performance in effected individuals. Staging which attempts to delineate the illness trajectory into phases can be considered as another facet of neuroprogression.[24] This conceptual framework of mood disorders is illustrated in Figure 7.2.

Allostatic Load and Neuroprogression

Mood disorders are complex and multifactorial diseases with genetic and environmental factors contributing to the clinical expression. These can also be regarded as diatheses involving the cumulative build-up of allostatic states, in which physiological "wear and tear" described as "allostatic load (AL)" progressively increases as stressors and mood episodes occur over time.[25] Affective episodes acting as allostatic states generate a burden that is responsible for illness progression commonly seen in major mood disorders. AL may contribute to a better understanding of the disease process, particularly to susceptibility to drug and alcohol abuse, decline in psychosocial functioning, cognitive dysfunction and affliction with cardiovascular, metabolic and endocrine diseases. The patients exhibit shifts in key mediators of AL, for instance persistent dysregulation of the hypothalamic–pituitary–adrenal (HPA) axis, modified immune response with a continual proinflammatory state, increased damage due to the occurrence of oxidative stress and decreased neuronal survival as a result of withdrawal of neurotrophic support. Greater during the acute phases of the disease, these deleterious changes remain subthreshold even during remission and damage the CNS, as the elements of brain tissue are particularly vulnerable to the mediators of AL.[26] Whereas, the body attempts to maintain homeostatic balance in the presence of ever mounting stress, increasing AL overwhelms the compensatory mechanisms causing permanent damage to the brain and the peripheral organs. Figure 7.3 depicts how intermediary factors of AL act in an orchestrated harmful manner inflicting incremental damage to the whole body.

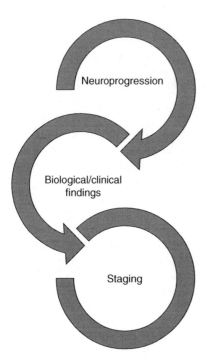

Figure 7.2 Linking neurobiological and clinical findings to neuroprogression and staging

Biological findings	Clinical findings
↑proinflammatory cytokines	↑episode severity
↑ROS	↑episode frequency
↓BDNF	↑suicidality
↓neurogenesis	↓cognitive performance
↑neuronal apoptosis	↓autonomy

BDNF – brain-derived neurotrophic factor; ROS – reactive oxygen species

Biomarkers of Mood Disorders

Potential Neuroimaging Markers

Many studies have reported the existence of changes in the brain structures of patients with both MDD and BD. Morphometric studies found enlargements of lateral and 3rd ventricles which were not evident from the onset of the disease and were often found only after several mood episodes. A study reported that the volume of the ventricles in BD patients during the first manic episode was similar to that of healthy individuals but lateral ventricles were 122% larger eight years after disease onset in cases with history of

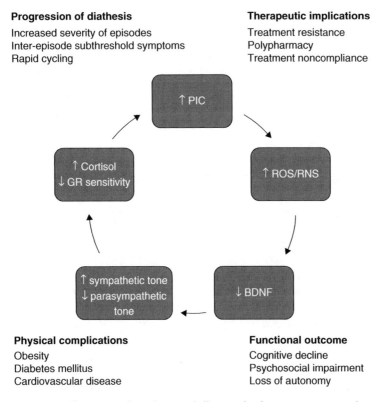

Progression of diathesis
Increased severity of episodes
Inter-episode subthreshold symptoms
Rapid cycling

Therapeutic implications
Treatment resistance
Polypharmacy
Treatment noncompliance

Physical complications
Obesity
Diabetes mellitus
Cardiovascular disease

Functional outcome
Cognitive decline
Psychosocial impairment
Loss of autonomy

Figure 7.3 The intermediary factors of allostatic load act in a vicious cycle in mood
disorders

BDNF – brain-derived neurotrophic factor; GR – glucocorticoid receptor; PIC – pro-inflammatory cytokines; RNS – reactive nitrogen species; ROS – reactive oxygen species

multiple affective episodes.[27] Other studies have found a progressive dimi-
nution in hippocampal volume in multiple episode patients. As hippocampal volume was normal at disease outset and decreased only after repeated
episodes, this may be a state marker of MDD.[28] A number of studies have
also found a reduction in the volume of some areas of the prefrontal cortex.
One study found that although the volume of the prefrontal lobe of patients
with BD was similar to that of healthy individuals, there were differences
in volume of gray matter in both the right and left prefrontal cortex. Their
findings also showed that disease duration might be correlated with a smaller
volume of gray matter in the left inferior prefrontal cortex.[29] Finally, many
studies have documented the existence of white matter hyperintensities in
individuals with BD. The presence of these abnormalities in deep white matter is about 2.5 times more likely to be found in BD patients than in healthy
controls.[30] One study reported the number of total brain hyperintensities

increased with the number of manic episodes.[31] A well-cited meta-analysis suggested that these lesions should be used as trait markers because white matter hyperintensities were frequent findings in family members who did not have BD.[32] As a concluding note, it must be mentioned that machine learning algorithms are being developed in earnest, with structural MRI as the basis, to help in the differential diagnosis and management of major mood disorders.

Brain-Derived Neurotrophic Factor

Neurotrophic factors are essential for neuronal differentiation and survival and play a vital role in dendritic growth, synaptogenesis and processes like long-term potentiation. BDNF is highly concentrated in limbic and paralimbic areas; it is generally believed that serum BDNF levels correlate with brain BDNF concentrations, so that peripheral fluctuations are a sensitive marker of disease activity. A recent meta-analysis indicates BD patients in the manic or depressive phase have lower blood concentrations of BDNF than healthy individuals, and that serum BDNF levels in euthymic patients are not significantly different from those found in controls.[33] Reduction in serum BDNF level may be a potential biomarker of acute episodes and could differentiate patients in a manic or depressive state from those in a euthymic phase at a sensitivity of 90% and a specificity of 85%.[34] In addition, another study found that laboratory measurements of serum BDNF concentrations may distinguish bipolar from unipolar depression at a diagnostic accuracy of 88% for values equal to or lower than 0.26 pg/ml. The authors compared plasma BDNF concentrations of BD patients in a depressive state with unipolar depression cases, and found that the first group expressed lower levels of BDNF. Clinically, the difference between bipolar and unipolar depression remains challenging, since BD can only be diagnosed with a history of a manic or hypomanic episode. Therefore, serum BDNF concentrations may be an important marker in the differential diagnosis of the two conditions.[35] Other studies suggest BDNF may be a biomarker of disease progression and severity. In this respect, BDNF values are inversely correlated with episode severity in MDD and BD cases. To explore the potential of blood BDNF to discriminate advanced and initial BD states, researchers showed that serum BDNF concentrations may discriminate patients with BD for less than three years from patients who have had the disease for over 10 years, at a sensitivity of 100%, specificity of 88% and accuracy of 95% for values equal to or lower than 0.62 pg/ml.[36] Another possible use of serum BDNF concentrations is the prediction of response to treatment and the assessment of pharmacological efficacy. In this regard, studies have found there is an increase and normalization of blood BDNF levels after appropriate treatment of acute mood episodes. Therefore, it is fair to conclude that serum BDNF is a promising marker of mood disorders and further research is likely to validate its use in clinical practice.[37]

Oxidative Stress

Oxidative stress is the result of imbalance between pro and antioxidants which results in the generation of an increased quantity of free radicals, such as reactive oxygen and nitrogen species (ROS and RNS). The latter produce cellular damage by reacting with macromolecules such as lipids, proteins, carbohydrates and DNA. The CNS is particularly vulnerable to oxidative injury, because the brain uses a great amount of oxygen which promotes the formation of ROS and RNS, and additionally has a limited antioxidant capacity. Glutathione is the main antioxidant in the brain, while the enzymes composing the antioxidant system are most importantly, superoxide dismutase (SOD), catalase (CAT) and glutathione peroxidase. The role of oxidative stress in the pathophysiology of mood disorders has been investigated in several studies, which consistently report changes in antioxidant enzymes, lipid peroxidation and free radical damage to the DNA. A meta-analysis concluded that some of the oxidative stress markers were elevated in plasma or blood cells of individuals with BD, particularly nitric oxide and thiobarbituric acid reactive substances (TBARS).[38] The analysis of blood TBARS (markers of lipid peroxidation) concentrations in patients with BD revealed that these were increased during all stages of the disease. This suggested that lipid damage occurred all along the course of BD and, therefore, serum levels of TBARS could be used as biomarkers of progression with the caveat that these showed increase with illness duration.[39] In addition, concentrations of nitric oxide were also elevated in BD, regardless of the mood state, and levels of 3-nitrotyrosine, another oxidative stress marker, were raised in the initial stages of the disorder.

One of the consequences of oxidative stress is DNA damage, and studies in patients with mood disorders have shown an increase in the frequency of this phenomenon. In BD cases, a study described a positive correlation between manic and depressive symptom severity and enhanced DNA damage.[40] In this vein, DNA damage has also been associated with reductions in telomere length in lymphocytes of individuals with mood disorders which is indicative of cumulative oxidative stress. Moreover, a study in patients with BD concluded that the number of shortened telomeres and mean telomere length were associated with the number of depressive episodes along life, and association with anxiety spectrum disorders contributed to the risk.[41] Telomere shortening physiologically occurs after each cell division as part of normal aging. However, telomere shortening found in individuals with mood disorders seems to be indicative of aging acceleration of the magnitude of about 10 years. These data may explain the connection between affective illnesses and early onset of medical comorbidities in this group of patients.

Another element to support the role of oxidative stress in mood disorders is the evidence that antioxidant compounds, such as N-acetylcysteine (NAC), are beneficial in the treatment of these conditions. NAC, a glutathione precursor, efficiently reduces depressive symptoms in patients with BD and improves their functioning and quality of life. Treatment effects of mood stabilizers seem to be associated with their action upon oxidative stress pathways. Patients with BD treated with lithium have a significant reduction of TBARS concentrations and of the SOD/CAT ratio, whereas healthy individuals exposed to lithium do not have the same changes. This may be secondary to lithium's inhibition of an important enzyme of the human kinome, namely GSK3β, with consequent antioxidant effects favorable for the treatment of BD.[42] Lastly, to evaluate systemic toxicity in mood disorders a study compared the concentrations of several markers in patients with BD, healthy individuals and patients with sepsis. One of their notable findings was the impressive scale of oxidative damage during acute episodes, which in some cases was as high as the level seen in patients with sepsis.[43] In view of the importance of peripheral oxidative stress markers, there is a need for further work so that these could be used in day-to-day clinical practice.

Inflammatory Factors

Inflammatory factors, i.e., cytokines, are proteins or glycoproteins secreted by cells of the immune system in response to noxious stimuli. Cytokines gain access to the CNS via the periphery, while microglia, the resident brain macrophages, also secrete these mediators. Proinflammatory cytokines like tumor necrosis factor-alpha (TNF-α) bind to neuronal death receptors and recruit Fas (first apoptosis signal) to activate caspase 8, a pro-apoptotic enzyme, leading to cell death. In mood disorder patients with repeated episodes, the increased neuronal loss via apoptosis has been documented as decrease in hippocampal volume and reduction in prefrontal gray matter.[44] Recent studies in both MDD and BD have confirmed the presence of a chronic inflammatory state. In general, affective episodes may be considered as proinflammatory states; for example, one study revealed that patients with a manic exacerbation had higher interleukin-2 (IL-2), IL-4 and IL-6 concentrations than controls, whereas patients with bipolar depression showed elevated levels of IL-6 only. During euthymic periods only IL-4 levels were raised, suggesting that mania and to a lesser degree depression was associated with a proinflammatory state.[45] Another study found that patients in a manic state had significantly higher concentrations of IL-6, TNF-α and high-sensitivity C-reactive protein (hs-CRP) than individuals without BD. After six weeks of treatment with mood stabilizing drugs, the same patients had decreased levels of these inflammatory indicators. However, hs-CRP values correlated significantly with reduction in manic symptomatology, suggesting this was the most consistent indicator of treatment response.[46]

At the same time, preliminary studies have found inflammatory biomarkers are capable of discriminating mood disorder patients in the initial phases of the disease from those in advanced stages. According to one study at advanced BD stages serum IL-10 concentrations (an anti-inflammatory cytokine) decreased and plasma TNF-α levels increased significantly. Another study found that when TNF-α concentrations were equal to or greater than

20.36 pg/ml, patients with BD at advanced stages could be discriminated from patients in initial stages at an accuracy of 91% and sensitivity and specificity of 97% and 85% respectively, indicating that TNF-α might be a potential biomarker of BD progression.[47] Increased concentrations of proinflammatory cytokines in mood disorders may indicate an association with high rates of medical comorbidities, particularly cardiovascular disease as these inflammatory changes may be risk factors for the development of obesity, hypertension, diabetes and atherosclerosis. In fact, medical burden is part of the early stages of major mood disorders as over 70% of young individuals are estimated to need treatment for chronic medical conditions. In contrast, middle-aged patients develop heart disease and hypertension at a younger age than adults without mood disorders, underscoring that medical burden should be included in the staging process.

Staging Models for Bipolar Disorder

Model Proposed by Berk et al.[48]

a) BD initiates with an asymptomatic phase (stage 0), which is directly connected to specific risk factors, for example family history of the illness and substance abuse.

b) Stage 1 is divided into 1a and 1b, characterized by the presence of mild, nonspecific mood symptoms, with the possibility of evolving to prodromal patterns.

c) Stage 2 is where the first episode takes place, in either the manic or depressive phase – the latter being more common.

d) Stage 3, divided into three phases, is characterized by the first relapse or the persistence of subclinical symptoms (phase 3a), an illness course with borderline symptoms (3b), or a remitting and recurring pattern (3c).

e) Finally, stage 4 refers to patients who do not achieve full remission of symptoms or are refractory to treatment.

Staging Model of Kapczinski et al.[49]

This model shifts the emphasis to functioning in the inter-episode as a means to stage defining BD, along with the characterization of biomarkers for each phase.

a) The patients are classified into five stages, starting with a latent phase (stage 0) in which individuals may experience mood and anxiety symptoms without overt presence of BD.

b) In stage 1, patients have already experienced an episode of mania or hypomania, but present adequate functioning and absence of cognitive deficits in the inter-episode.

c) In stage 2, subclinical symptoms, comorbidities and mild cognitive dysfunction are present in the inter-episode.

d) In stage 3, patients present with marked cognitive and functional impairment.

e) Finally, stage 4 includes individuals with severe cognitive and functional impairment, leading to loss of autonomy.

Duffy's Model[50]

Duffy recently suggested a version of BD staging and according to this model patients would first be classified into either classical or bipolar spectrum disorders. Each group could then have the following possible stages:

a) Stage 0 or prodromal period in which patients are well but have a positive family history in 1st degree relatives.

b) Stage 1 occurring in children or adolescents is marked by anxiety, sleep and adjustment disorders which are of a severe nature in bipolar spectrum cases as compared to classical, lithium-responsive BD patients.

c) Stage 2, which again has onset in young adulthood, is characterized by well-defined and circumscribed mood episodes, chiefly of a depressive nature. However, in bipolar spectrum patients with history of psychosis in 1st degree relatives there could be deficit symptoms like amotivation, lack of affect and anhedonia.

d) Stage 3 is characterized by remitting manic and depressive episodes responsive to lithium in classical BD. In contrast, bipolar spectrum patients experience psychotic symptoms, cognitive deficits and psychosocial decline.

e) Stage 4 is marked by euphoric mania in classical BD, whereas there are mixed or psychotic manic symptoms in bipolar spectrum disorders.

f) The final stage in classical BD is characterized by some neuropsychiatric and medical comorbidities but the illness still remains responsive to lithium therapy and has an overall better prognosis. In contradistinction, the other group shows features reminiscent of schizophrenia spectrum disorders with positive psychotic symptoms, as well as cognitive decline and functional deterioration.

Staging Models for Major Depressive Disorder[51]

Recently Ferensztajn et al. put forward a staging model for MDD with its basis on the notions of allostatic load and neuroprogression.

a) According to the authors stage 1 is characterized by the preclinical phase in which there are such risk factors as positive family history of MDD in 1st degree relatives (1a), or there are nonspecific neuropsychiatric symptoms not achieving the level of major depressive episode (1b).

b) In stage 2 there is the occurrence of a major depressive episode but with complete remission of symptoms.

c) Stage 3 is characterized by ill-defined residual symptoms (3a), or dysthymia (3b) in the inter-episode.

d) Stage 4 is marked by recurrent major depressive episodes (4a), or "double depression" if dysthymia is present (4b), i.e., persistence of subthreshold depressive symptoms between episodes.

e) Stage 5 is where there is the presence of "chronic depression", i.e., the duration of depressive episode is for two years or longer.

Therapeutic Implications of Staging

In other fields of medicine staging is widely used to choose appropriate treatments and inform the prognosis. However, this is a new trend in psychiatry and only recently have the first models of staging of psychiatric disorders been developed. For staging designs to have investigative value, the course of the disease should be predictable along time, and the illness at the initial stages should be associated with simpler treatment requirements and a better outcome. In addition, treatment efficacy should also be greater in the beginning of the ailment and a subsequent progressive decline should be expected, culminating in treatment resistance. For this reason staging formats should to be constructed in parallel with treatment algorithms, as different stages have diverse therapeutic requirements. Therefore, it is presumed that staging is instrumental in choosing personalized optimal management plans, and is simultaneously helpful in making clear the prospects in individual cases. It must be understood that early interventions are essential in preventing the diathesis from advancing. While treatment during the initial stages should primarily focus on neuroprotective strategies, therapy during more advanced phases should be palliative and rehabilitative to control the consequences of disease progression. The importance assigned to neuroprotective approaches may take psychiatry to a new era of preventive medicine.

Limitations of the Staging Models

As far as the staging models for mood disorders are concerned the following points need to be highlighted:

1) A developmental clinical staging approach represents an important advance supporting earlier and more accurate psychiatric diagnosis.

2) Clinical staging of mood disorders must consider both the natural history and the heterogeneity of the diagnosis.

3) A comprehensive evidence-based staging model of affective illnesses is important to promote early detection and intervention, as well as identifying markers of illness predisposition and progression.

4) The proponents of staging affective disorders on the basis of neuroprogression and allostatic load have focused on differentiating earlier- from

later-stage illness in adult patients meeting full diagnostic criteria for the disorder.

5) These studies consider neither the evidence of early antecedent risk syndromes nor the developmental illness trajectory leading up to the diagnosis of BD or MDD, as reported in several large prospective studies of the offspring of parents with these conditions.

6) The proposed staging models should be examined with the caveat that these provide an aggregate view derived from research studies and will not apply to all high-risk offspring as environmental and epigenetic factors operate in the expression of the diathesis.

7) The problem with the allostatic load model (Kapczinsky et al.) is that it focuses solely on progression of end-stage established disease, rather than articulating a staging model based on the full natural history of illness evolution.

8) While Berk et al.'s approach is more comprehensive, it collapses numerous discrete early clinical stages of illness development into a single very heterogeneous stage 1. Further, it does not incorporate family history as a way to identifying high-risk individuals, although a positive family history is the most important risk factor predicting for at least classical BD. Without the context of positive family history, the early stages are too nonspecific and would yield a very high rate of false positives.

9) Finally, the staging models will need to be refined and informed by future research advances to be of heuristic value.

Conclusion

Staging of major psychiatric disorders is gaining momentum as the clinical significance of this framework is substantial. Several lines of research show that the course of major mood disorders follows a predictable and evolving path, from milder to progressively more severe presentations; staging models foster better understanding of the trajectory of these illnesses. While the blueprint of any staging system does not of necessity imply that patients would pass through each phase sequentially, it does give an aggregate view of how the illness unfolds as it develops. The extrapolative nature of the staging schema helps in formulating individually tailored treatment plans and defining prognosis. Appropriate and adequate treatment in the early phases should prevent advancement to the latter periods in which lasting damage has, in essence, occurred. In susceptible individuals with an ultra-high risk profile, interventions in the earliest stages give an opportunity to prevent the ailment from progressing and resulting in a whole host of undesirable sequelae. Each one of the existing staging models has its merits and limitations, but unquestionably there is a great need for this proposal. It is expected that future research will lead to refinements in the staging protocols with better outcomes for people with mood disorders, which indeed are intractable conditions with poor prospects for many patients.

Summary Points

- In medicine, staging is widely used to delineate chronic, recalcitrant diseases.
- There is growing realization that major mood disorders are evolving conditions which have a prodrome, an active phase and a residual state.
- In adolescents and young adults mood disorders often start from non-specific antecedents, are characterized by well-circumscribed episodes in the early stages with progression to severe presentations accompanied by marked psychosocial impairments.
- The evolution alluded to here is foreseeable in a great majority of patients and family history brings important context in this regard.
- Researchers in the field have come forward with meticulous staging models of mood disorders which assist in predicting the course and outcome and help in the management of these difficult to treat conditions.
- This framework is conducive to understanding the illness trajectory, making individualized treatment plans and delivering personalized care to patients with mood disorders.
- On the other hand it paves the way for a more comprehensive know-how regarding the pathogenesis of these conditions, supports the identification of trait- and state-specific markers and the incorporation of these indicators in routine practice.
- The usefulness of the staging protocol is enormous and it is conceivable that further refinements in this area would make it an indispensable tool in the general management of patients.

References

1) Korf J. Delayed mood transitions in major depressive disorder. Med Hypotheses 2014;82:581–588.
2) Cosci F, Fava GA. Staging of mental disorders: systematic review. Psychother Psychosom 2013;82:20–34.
3) Zhang L, Yu X, Fang YR, Ungvari GS, Ng CH, Chiu HF, et al. Duration of untreated bipolar disorder: a multicenter study. Sci Rep 2017;7:44811.
4) Mwangi B, Wu MJ, Cao B, Passos IC, Lavagnino L, Keser Z, et al. Individualized prediction and clinical staging of bipolar disorders using neuroanatomical biomarkers. Biol Psychiatry CognNeurosci Neuroimaging 2016;1:186–194.
5) Slyepchenko A, Maes M, Köhler CA, Anderson G, Quevedo J, Alves GS, et al. T helper 17 cells may drive neuroprogression in major depressive disorder: proposal of an integrative model. Neurosci Biobehav Rev 2016;64:83–100.
6) Fernandes BS, Berk M. Staging in bipolar disorder: one step closer to precision psychiatry. Rev Bras Psiquiatr 2017;39:88–89.
7) Zivanovic O, Nedic A. Kraepelin's concept of manic-depressive insanity: one hundred years later. J Affect Disord 2012;137:15–24.
8) Passos IC, Kapczinski F. Should bipolar disorder treatment be modified depending on staging? Expert Rev Neurother 2017;17:93–95.

9) Duffy A, Horrocks J, Doucette S, Keown-Stoneman C, McCloskey S, Grof P. The developmental trajectory of bipolar disorder. Br J Psychiatry 2014;204:122–128.

10) Duffy A, Horrocks J, Doucette S, Keown-Stoneman C, McCloskey S, Grof P. Childhood anxiety: an early predictor of mood disorders in offspring of bipolar parents. J Affect Disord 2013;150:363–369.

11) Garnham J, Munro A, Slaney C, Macdougall M, Passmore M, Duffy A, et al. Prophylactic treatment response in bipolar disorder: results of a naturalistic observation study. J Affect Disord 2007;104:185–190.

12) Duffy A, Alda M, Milin R, Grof P. A consecutive series of treated affected offspring of parents with bipolar disorder: is response associated with the clinical profile? Can J Psychiatry 2007;52:369–376.

13) Vedel Kessing L, Vradi E, Kragh Andersen P. Diagnostic stability in pediatric bipolar disorder. J Affect Disord;172:417–421.

14) Goldstein BI, Lotrich F, Axelson DA, Gill MK, Hower H, Goldstein TR, et al. Inflammatory markers among adolescents and young adults with bipolar spectrum disorders. J Clin Psychiatry 2015;76:1556–1563.

15) Sparks GM, Axelson DA, Yu H, Ha W, Ballester J, Diler RS, et al. Disruptive mood dysregulation disorder and chronic irritability in youth at familial risk for bipolar disorder. J Am Acad Child Adolesc Psychiatry 2014;53:408–416.

16) Kim JW, Yu H, Ryan ND, Axelson DA, Goldstein BI, Goldstein TR, et al. Longitudinal trajectories of ADHD symptomatology in offspring of parents with bipolar disorder and community controls. J Clin Psychiatry 2015;76:599–606.

17) Goldstein BI, Shamseddeen W, Axelson DA, Kalas C, Monk K, Brent DA, et al. Clinical, demographic, and familial correlates of bipolar spectrum disorders among offspring of parents with bipolar disorder. J Am Acad Child Adolesc Psychiatry 2010;49:388–396.

18) Faedda GL, Serra G, Marangoni C, Salvatore P, Sani G, Vázquez GH, et al. Clinical risk factors for bipolar disorders: a systematic review of prospective studies. J Affect Disord 2014;168:314–321.

19) Duffy A, Alda M, Hajek T, Sherry SB, Grof P. Early stages in the development of bipolar disorder. J Affect Disord 2010;121:127–135.

20) Sara GE, Malhi GS. Trends in diagnosis of bipolar disorder: Have the boundaries changed? Aust N Z J Psychiatry 2015;49:1021–1028.

21) Duffy A, Malhi GS, Grof P. Do the trajectories of bipolar disorder and schizophrenia follow a universal staging model? Can J Psychiatry 2017;62:115–122.

22) Moylan S, Maes M, Wray NR, Berk M. The neuroprogressive nature of major depressive disorder: pathways to disease evolution and resistance, and therapeutic implications. Mol Psychiatry 2013;18:595–606.

23) Kapczinski NS, Mwangi B, Cassidy RM, Librenza-Garcia D, Bermudez MB, Kauer-Sant'anna M, et al. Neuroprogression and illness trajectories in bipolar disorder. Expert Rev Neurother 2017;17:277–285.

24) Gama CS, Kunz M, Magalhães PV, Kapczinski F. Staging and neuroprogression in bipolar disorder: a systematic review of the literature. Rev Bras Psiquiatr 2013;35:70–74.

25) McEwen BS. Biomarkers for assessing population and individual health and disease related to stress and adaptation. Metabolism 2015;64:S2-S10.

26) Walker AJ, Kim Y, Price JB, Kale RP, McGillivray JA, Berk M, et al. Stress, inflammation, and cellular vulnerability during early stages of affective disorders: biomarker strategies and opportunities for prevention and intervention. Front Psychiatry 2014;5:34.

27) Quigley SJ, Scanlon C, Kilmartin L, Emsell L, Langan C, Hallahan B, et al. Volume and shape analysis of subcortical brain structures and ventricles in euthymic bipolar I disorder. Psychiatry Res 2015;233:324–330.

28) Colle R, Chupin M, Cury C, Vandendrie C, Gressier F, Hardy P, et al. Depressed suicide attempters have smaller hippocampus than depressed patients without suicide attempts. J Psychiatr Res 2015;61:13–18.

29) Savitz JB, Price JL, Drevets WC. Neuropathological and neuromorphometric abnormalities in bipolar disorder: view from the medial prefrontal cortical network. Neurosci Biobehav Rev 2014;42:132–147.

30) Tighe SK, Reading SA, Rivkin P, Caffo B, Schweizer B, Pearlson G, et al. Total white matter hyperintensity volume in bipolar disorder patients and their healthy relatives. Bipolar Disord 2002;14:888–893.

31) Kieseppä T, Mäntylä R, Tuulio-Henriksson A, Luoma K, Mantere O, Ketokivi M, et al. White matter hyperintensities and cognitive performance in adult patients with bipolar I, bipolar II, and major depressive disorders. Eur Psychiatry 2014;29:226–232.

32) Beyer JL, Young R, Kuchibhatla M, Krishnan KR. Hyperintense MRI lesions in bipolar disorder: a meta-analysis and review. Int Rev Psychiatry 2009;21:394–409.

33) Fernandes BS, Molendijk ML, Köhler CA, Soares JC, Leite CM, Machado-Vieira R, et al. Peripheral brain-derived neurotrophic factor (BDNF) as a biomarker in bipolar disorder: a meta-analysis of 52 studies. BMC Med 2015;13:289.

34) Fernandes BS, Gama CS, Ceresér KM, Yatham LN, Fries GR, Colpo G, et al. Brain-derived neurotrophic factor as a state-marker of mood episodes in bipolar disorders: a systematic review and meta-regression analysis. J Psychiatr Res 2011;45:995–1004.

35) Fernandes BS, Gama CS, Kauer-Sant'Anna M, Lobato MI, Belmonte-de-Abreu P, Kapczinski F. Serum brain-derived neurotrophic factor in bipolar and unipolar depression: a potential adjunctive tool for differential diagnosis. J Psychiatr Res 2009;43:1200–1204.

36) Kapczinski F, Fernandes BS, Kauer-Sant'Anna M, Gama CS, Yatham LN, Berk M. The concept of staging in bipolar disorder: the role of BDNF and TNF-alpha as biomarkers. Acta Neuropsychiatr 2009;21:272–274.

37) Huang TL, Lin CC. Advances in biomarkers of major depressive disorder. Adv Clin Chem 2015;68:177–204.

38) Brown NC, Andreazza AC, Young LT. An updated meta-analysis of oxidative stress markers in bipolar disorder. Psychiatry Res 2014;218:61–68.

39) Siwek M, Sowa-Kucma M, Styczen K, Misztak P, Szewczyk B, Topor-Madry R, et al. Thiobarbituric acid-reactive substances: markers of an acute episode and a late stage of bipolar disorder. Neuropsychobiology 2016;73:116–122.

40) Jacoby AS, Vinberg M, Poulsen HE, Kessing LV, Munkholm K. T Increased DNA and RNA damage by oxidation in patients with bipolar I disorder. Thiobarbituric acid-reactive substances: markers of an acute episode and a late stage of bipolar disorder. Transl Psychiatry 2016;6:e867.

41) Lima IM, Barros A, Rosa DV, Albuquerque M, Malloy-Diniz L, Neves FS, et al. Analysis of telomere attrition in bipolar disorder. J Affect Disord 2015;172:43–47.

42) Wada A. Lithium and neuropsychiatric therapeutics: neuroplasticity via glycogen synthase kinase-3beta, beta-catenin, and neurotrophin cascades. J PharmacolSci 2009;110:14–28.

43) Kapczinski F, Dal-Pizzol F, Teixeira AL, Magalhaes PV, Kauer-Sant'Anna M, Klamt F, et al. A systemic toxicity index developed to assess peripheral changes in mood episodes. Mol Psychiatry 2010;15:784–786.

44) Kim YK, Na KS. Application of machine learning classification for structural brain MRI in mood disorders: Critical review from a clinical perspective. Prog Neuropsychopharmacol Biol Psychiatry 2017;[Epub ahead of print].

45) Luo Y, He H, Zhang M, Huang X, Fan N. Altered serum levels of TNF-α, IL-6 and IL-18 in manic, depressive, mixed state of bipolar disorder patients. Psychiatry Res 2016;244:19–23.

46) Uyanik V, Tuglu C, Gorgulu Y, Kunduracilar H, Uyanik MS. Assessment of cyto-kine levels and hs-CRP in bipolar I disorder before and after treatment. Psychiatry Res 2015;228:386–392.

47) Doganavsargil-Baysal O, Cinemre B, Aksoy UM, Akbas H, Metin O, Fettahoglu C, et al. Levels of TNF-α, soluble TNF receptors (sTNFR1, sTNFR2), and cogni-tion in bipolar disorder. Hum Psychopharmacol. 2013;28:160–167.

48) Berk M, Berk L, Dodd S, Cotton S, Macneil C, Daglas R, et al. Stage managing bipolar disorder. Bipolar Disord 2014;16:471–477.

49) Kapczinski F, Dias VV, Kauer-Sant'Anna M, Frey BN, Grassi-Oliveira R, Colom F, et al. Clinical implications of a staging model for bipolar disorders. Expert Rev Neurother 2009;9:957–66.

50) Duffy A. Toward a comprehensive clinical staging model for bipolar disorder: inte-grating the evidence. Can J Psychiatry 2014;59:659–666.

51) Ferensztajn E, Remlinger-Molenda A, Rybakowski J. Staging of unipolar affective illness. Psychiatr Pol 2014;48:1127–1141.

8   The Management of Treatment-Resistant Depression

Monoamines and Beyond

Introduction

Major depressive disorder (MDD) is an important cause of disability worldwide with significant impact on patients' functioning and quality of life. Standard antidepressants are only effective for approximately one-third of MDD patients, as measured by remission, indicated by a score ≤ 7 on the 17-item Hamilton Rating Scale for Depression (HRSD). Furthermore, after multiple antidepressant trials, approximately one-third of patients still remain treatment resistant with substantial functional impairments. These figures are extrapolated from the results of the STAR*D (Sequenced Treatment Alternatives to Relieve Depression) trial, a very comprehensive and large clinical study on MDD.[1] Treatment-resistant depression (TRD) is therefore a subject of high relevance as it seriously affects a significant proportion of MDD patients. While several definitions and staging models for TRD have been suggested, here this term will be used to broadly refer to an insufficient response to a single adequate trial of a first-line antidepressant. Of note, there is a lack of consensus on a unified definition of TRD, which is a limiting factor for progress in the field of MDD therapeutics.[2] Figure 8.1 gives a schematic representation of the phenomenon of TRD and illustrates that approximately 33% of patients with MDD remain symptomatic even after multiple trials of antidepressant medications.

Switching or Combining First-Line Antidepressants

Once a patient fails to respond to an adequate trial of a standard antidepressant, the next step to consider is switching or combining these agents, although there is equivocal evidence for either strategy.

Switching

After a first selective serotonin reuptake inhibitor (SSRI) trial, switching within or between antidepressant classes may be an effective approach. Switching the antidepressant from one class to another is a common tactic

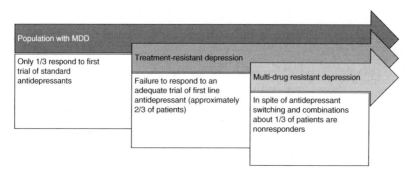

Figure 8.1 The phenomenon of treatment-resistant depression

Major depressive disorder is a heterogeneous condition and shows varied response to standard antidepressants. Large scale trials like STAR*D have revealed remission, as measured by a validated scale like the Hamilton Rating Scale for Depression, is only achieved in one-third of patients with the first trial of a standard antidepressant. Even after employing switching strategies and drug combinations, about 33% of the patients still are unable to achieve a response with the currently available antidepressant medications. This situation implies that targets other than monoamines must be explored to bring adequate relief to people with MDD.

with support in the literature, though there is evidence suggesting this strategy is not superior to switching within classes.

Venlafaxine and duloxetine are serotonin and norepinephrine reuptake inhibitors (SNRIs) widely used for depression and anxiety disorders. After the failure of an SSRI, substituting these drugs may be a more useful policy when compared to swapping SSRIs. A randomized, double-blind trial (RCT) enrolling 122 patients showed switching to venlafaxine yielded a remission rate of 42% compared with 20% for paroxetine (*p*=0.01).[3] Another RCT in a larger sample (n=406), however, found no significant difference in venlafaxine extended-release (XR) versus citalopram to treat TRD. A secondary analysis showed in more severe MDD (HRSD-21 score ≥ 31), venlafaxine XR performed better than citalopram in improving depressive symptoms.[4] In an open-label study (n=3097), a relatively small but significant superiority of venlafaxine XR over other antidepressants (mostly SSRIs or mirtazapine) was demonstrated; the remission rate in the venlafaxine group was 59.3% versus 51.5% in the comparison group.[5] In STAR*D (n=727), however, remission rates with venlafaxine XR treatment (24.8%) were not significantly superior than remission rates with bupropion sustained release (SR), a dopamine-norepinephrine reuptake inhibitor (21.3%), or with sertraline (18.1%). Notably, evidence from several meta-analyses back the superiority of SNRIs over SSRIs, especially in severe MDD.

Mirtazapine, a noradrenergic, specific serotonergic antidepressant, is an antagonist of receptors α-2, 5-HT2 and 5-HT3, and agonist of postsynaptic 5-HT1A receptors. Although both mirtazapine and venlafaxine possess a dual action profile, mirtazapine achieved inferior remission rates than venlafaxine after an initial antidepressant failure in the ARGOS open-label study (n=3097). In the STAR*D study, 235 patients who had two antidepressant failures were randomized to mirtazapine or nortryptiline; mirtazapine was not significantly different from nortryptiline regarding remission rates (12.3% versus 19.8%, respectively).

Agomelatine is a drug that works through melatonergic agonism (on MT1 and MT2 receptors) and 5-HT2C antagonism. Agomelatine has been shown to be efficacious in MDD in several studies. Yet, there is no evidence of agomelatine's efficacy, particularly in TRD, thus necessitating further studies.

In an open-label study, 92 patients with TRD received nortryptiline and showed response and remission rates of about 40% and 12%, respectively.[6] The comparison of switching to nortryptiline or mirtazapine after treatment failure showed no difference as previously discussed (STAR*D study). After a nonresponse with either sertraline (n=117) or imipramine (n=51), patients were assigned to a 12-week trial with the other medication and had nearly 50% of response on both switches.[7] Thus, swapping a SSRI for a tricyclic antidepressant (TCA) or the other way around is perhaps a good policy in TRD, as there is support for this strategy in the literature.

The STAR*D study evaluated 109 patients who received venlafaxine plus mirtazapine or tranylcypromine after three consecutive trial failures. The study found low remission rates in both groups – tranylcypromine (6.9%) and venlafaxine plus mirtazapine (13.7%) – with no significant difference. Notably, mean dose in the tranylcypromine group was relatively low (36.9 mg/day) and almost half of the patients on tranylcypromine had less than six weeks of treatment, which significantly marred the interpretation of the outcomes.[8] In two controlled, partial crossover studies involving MDD subjects who had undergone at least two unsuccessful TCA trials, 47 patients were assigned to tranylcypromine, which was effective in around 50% of them. However, the small sample size and the design of the studies restricted the interpretation of this conclusion.

Antidepressants in Combination

An open-label study enrolled 225 patients with TRD treated with paroxetine augmented with other drugs. After eight weeks of add-on treatment to paroxetine, remission was achieved by 32.6% of the patients with buspirone and 42.6% with trazodone; the difference between the groups was not significant.[9] Reboxetine add-on to duloxetine in MDD patients who did not respond to an eight-week duloxetine trial was evaluated in an open-label study; 76% of the patients on 12 weeks reboxetine augmentation responded, and 69.3% remitted.

In a four-week RCT of antidepressant augmentation with mirtazapine, adjunctive mirtazapine produced a significantly superior response rate of 63.6% versus 20% for the placebo. Two RCTs found that in MDD patients with and without TRD, mirtazapine in combination with a SSRI, bupropion, or venlafaxine was superior to either agent alone.[10,11] Consistently, a meta-analysis in MDD not just restricted to TRD showed that mirtazapine combination to SSRI was superior to a SSRI alone (RR=1.88, 95% CI, 1.06–3.33).[12]

However, as reported above, in the STAR*D study MDD patients receiving a combination of mirtazapine plus venlafaxine after three treatment failures had a remission rate of only 13.7%. Moreover, in a single-blind, 12-week study with 665 patients with severe or recurrent MDD, similar remission (37.7%–38.9%) and response (57.4%–59.4%) rates were found among the three study groups: mirtazapine (up to 45 mg/day) plus venlafaxine XR (up to 300 mg/day), escitalopram (up to 20 mg/day) plus placebo, and bupropion SR (up to 400 mg/day) plus escitalopram. Also, at the long-term follow-up of seven months, remission rates (41.8%–46.6%), response rates (57.4%–59.4%) and most secondary outcomes were not significantly different.[13] One meta-analysis (Rocha et al., reference 12 below) assessing the efficacy of antidepressant combinations in MDD found that a TCA plus SSRI was superior to the SSRI alone in achieving both remission (RR=8.58, 95% CI=1.70–43.32) and response (RR=1.78, 95% CI=1.07–2.93). More studies are needed to establish the best combinations for TRD.

Combining Atypical Antipsychotics With Standard Antidepressants

Atypical antipsychotics (AAP) are able to modulate dopaminergic system and monoamine reuptake, with several agents also showing 5-HT2 receptors antagonism and blockade of α2-adrenergic receptors. Two meta-analyses of placebo-controlled trials have demonstrated that adjunctive AAP is an effective approach in the treatment of TRD, with a number needed to treat of nearly nine. The evidence for specific AAP agents approved by the United States Food and Drug Administration (FDA) for the combination treatment of MDD is summarized below.

Brexpiprazole

This drug, structurally related to aripiprazole, is a serotonin-dopamine activity modulator. In July 2015 it received FDA approval for schizophrenia and augmentation therapy of MDD. It shows partial agonism at the D2 receptor and possibly functional selectivity at this site. Compared to aripiprazole, brexpiprazole has lower intrinsic activity at the D2R, but exhibits 10-fold higher affinity at the 5-HT1A receptor where it acts as a partial agonist. Two recently published phase III trials investigated the potential of brexpiprazole as an augmentation agent in TRD. The two identically designed studies included subjects who had inadequate response to one to three standard antidepressants (AD) for their current depressive episode. All patients entered a prospective eight-week phase of open-label antidepressant therapy and those who failed to sufficiently respond were randomized to AD + brexpiprazole or AD + placebo and followed in a double-blind fashion for a total of six weeks. The primary outcome measure was change in Montgomery-Asberg Depression Rating Scale (MADRS) from baseline to week 6. In the first study brexpiprazole 3 mg/day was superior to placebo on MADRS total score (-8.29 versus -6.33; $p = 0.0079$), but brexpiprazole 1 mg/day failed to separate from placebo (-7.64 versus -6.33; $p = 0.0737$). In the second study, brexpiprazole 2 mg/day showed superior efficacy over placebo in changes from baseline to week 6 on MADRS total scores (-8.36 versus -5.15; $p = 0.0002$). Further, the active agent was also better than placebo on the Sheehan Disability Scale (-1.35 versus -0.89; $p = 0.0349$). The most common treatment-related adverse events were weight gain (brexpiprazole, 8%; placebo, 3.1%) and akathisia (7.4% versus 1.0%). Taken as a whole, brexpiprazole in addition to standard antidepressants was safe and well tolerated in the two phase III RCTs.[14]

Aripiprazole

This third generation antipsychotic, first introduced in 2002 for schizophrenia, is well studied as an adjunctive therapy in MDD. With regards to controlled studies, three matching RCTs showed aripiprazole augmentation of traditional antidepressants was statistically superior to placebo in MDD patients who were nonresponders to one to three adequate antidepressant trials. A post hoc analysis of the abovementioned three RCTs divided patients into two categories – in one group were minimal-improvers on antidepressant monotherapy after 6–8 weeks of administration and in the second batch were non-improvers as defined by the Clinical Global Impression-Improvement (CGI-I) scale. After six weeks of adjunctive aripiprazole or placebo the remission rates were higher for the active drug in both groups (minimal-improvers – 38.8% versus 26.6%, $p < 0.05$; non-improvers – 24.0% versus 10.3%, $p < 0.05$). The most common adverse events with add-on aripiprazole were akathisia, restlessness and insomnia.[15] Another pooled analysis of the same RCTs stratified patients according to baseline MADRS scores as follows: mild ≤ 24; moderate $= 25$–30; severe ≥ 31. The results showed aripiprazole produced greater improvement than placebo in the MADRS scores regardless of MDD severity at baseline. A third post hoc analysis investigated the efficacy of adjunctive aripiprazole in MDD patients whose symptoms worsened with antidepressant monotherapy. In the prospective, open-label phase 106 subjects out of 1065 antidepressant monotherapy nonresponders actually deteriorated as assessed by MADRS. Those cases who worsened showed higher response and remission rates with aripiprazole compared to placebo during the six-week double-blind part of the studies (36.6% versus 22.5% and 25.4% versus 12.4%, respectively). Similarly, aripiprazole was superior to placebo for the 905 subjects who did not show deterioration on antidepressant monotherapy.[16]

Quetiapine

This second generation antipsychotic has been well studied in MDD, both as monotherapy and adjunctively to first-line antidepressants. In this context the first RCT was published in 2007, in which quetiapine augmentation of SSRI/venlafaxine was compared to placebo in a small group of MDD patients (N = 58) with comorbid anxiety (Hamilton Anxiety Rating Scale [HAM-A] ≥ 14) and residual depressive symptoms (Clinical Global Impression-Severity [CGI-S] ≥ 4). The mean change in HRSD and HAM-A total scores from baseline to study endpoint (week 8) was significantly greater with quetiapine (average dose 182 mg/day) than placebo (-11.2 versus -5.5, p = 0.008; -12.5 versus -5.9, p = 0.002, respectively). The onset of quetiapine efficacy (HRSD/HAM-A/CGI-S) was rapid by week 1 and continued through to week 8. Response, defined as ≥ 50% decrease in baseline HRSD scores, was numerically but not significantly higher for quetiapine than placebo. Similarly, remission rate (HRSD total scores ≤ 7) was also higher for the active agent (31% versus 17%) but this difference did not reach statistical significance. Adverse events for quetiapine were in line with its known side effect profile, and sedation and somnolence were most frequently reported. In conclusion, quetiapine was shown to be effective as augmentation of SSRI/venlafaxine therapy in patients with major depression, comorbid anxiety and residual depressive symptoms, with no unexpected tolerability issues.[17] The efficacy of quetiapine XR augmentation was shown in two similarly designed (150, 300 mg/day and placebo) six-week RCTs (N = 936). In both trials, the primary endpoint was mean changes in MADRS total score from baseline. In these studies quetiapine XR was statistically superior to placebo on the primary efficacy measure and this change was evident from week 1.

Quetiapine XR monotherapy has been studied in several short-term RCTs in MDD, both in fixed or flexible dose designs. In the majority of these trials, the active drug showed superiority over placebo on such validated efficacy measures as the MADRS. The dose of quetiapine XR was up to a maximum of 300 mg/day and trial durations varied from 6–8 weeks; the active agent separated from placebo as early as week 1 and this superiority was maintained until the end of the study period. The most common adverse events associated with quetiapine XR were dry mouth, sedation and somnolence. Extrapyramidal side effects were distinctly uncommon, but metabolic changes like increased serum glucose and lipids were more often observed.[18] In conclusion:

1) Quetiapine alone or adjunctively to standard antidepressants has valid efficacy in the treatment of nonpsychotic MDD.
2) In patients with MDD with psychotic features, quetiapine in conjunction with first-line antidepressants is superior to antidepressant monotherapy.
3) Quetiapine augmentation is a convincing option in TRD.
4) It has value in MDD with comorbid conditions like anxiety and fibromyalgia.

5) It is effective across such demographic variables as age, gender and race.
6) The medication has valid efficacy in MDD regardless of such illness factors as severity, duration and number of depressive episodes.
7) The effective dose in MDD is from 100 to 300 mg/day which is less than the maximum recommended dose of 600 mg/day in schizophrenia.
8) There is a caveat, it has the potential to cause metabolic abnormalities and careful monitoring is warranted in this regard.

Olanzapine/Fluoxetine

Adjunctive olanzapine has been studied in at least four RCTs in TRD and specifically olanzapine/fluoxetine combination (OFC) has been compared to both placebo and active comparators. A pooled analysis of these studies showed that OFC had clearly demonstrated significantly greater improvements in MADRS (primary efficacy measure) total score than fluoxetine or olanzapine alone and also resulted in higher remission rates. The short-term efficacy of OFC for treatment-resistant depression was supported by these trials.[19] In a more recently published long-term trial of up to 27 weeks, relapse rates were compared for fluoxetine monotherapy and OFC in stabilized patients on the combination treatment. Time to relapse was significantly longer in the OFC group than in the fluoxetine monotherapy group ($p < 0.001$). Additionally, with regards to safety no significant differences emerged between treatment groups in terms of adverse events ($p = 0.621$). However, the rate of patients who experienced clinically significant (> 7%) weight gain was greater for OFC than fluoxetine (11.8% and 2.3% respectively; $p < 0.001$). At the endpoint, the mean differences were significant for weight gain (OFC +1.14 kg, fluoxetine -2.78 kg; $p < 0.001$).[20] Finally, it must be mentioned that OFC is not only FDA approved in treatment-resistant unipolar depression, but it also has this endorsement for depressive episodes in bipolar I disorder.

Vortioxetine in Treatment-Resistant Depression

Vortioxetine is a new multimodal antidepressant approved for the treatment of MDD as monotherapy. It is a 5-HT3, 5-HT7 and 5-HT1D receptor antagonist, 5-HT1B receptor partial agonist, 5-HT1A receptor agonist and serotonin (5-HT) transporter (SERT) inhibitor. Vortioxetine increases serotonergic, noradrenergic, dopaminergic, cholinergic, histaminergic and glutamatergic neurotransmission in brain structures associated with MDD. These multiple effects likely derive from its interaction with 5-HT-receptor-mediated negative feedback mechanisms regulating neuronal activity. Preclinical animal models reveal differences from SSRIs and SNRIs, including antidepressant-like activity, increased synaptic plasticity and improved cognitive function. Vortioxetine had clinical efficacy in patients with MDD: 11 placebo-controlled studies (including one in elderly people) with efficacy in eight (seven positive, one supportive), one positive active comparator study plus a positive relapse prevention study. In two positive studies, vortioxetine was superior to placebo in pre-defined cognitive outcome measures. The clinically effective dose range (5–20 mg/day) spans ~ 50% to > 80% SERT occupancy. SERT and 5-HT3 receptors are primarily occupied at 5 mg, while at 20 mg, all targets are likely occupied at functionally relevant levels. The side effect profile is similar to that of SSRIs, with gastrointestinal symptoms being most common, and a low incidence of sexual dysfunction and sleep disruption possibly ascribed to vortioxetine's unique receptor modulation.[21]

A review of the extant literature revealed three studies in which MDD patients were switched from SSRI/SNRI therapy to vortioxetine due to lack of efficacy or tolerability. Vortioxetine was evaluated versus agomelatine directly (REVIVE) and versus sertraline, venlafaxine, bupropion and citalopram in an indirect treatment comparison (ITC) from switch studies retrieved in the literature review. Vortioxetine showed significant benefits over agomelatine on efficacy, functioning, and quality-of-life outcomes, with fewer withdrawals due to adverse events (AEs; REVIVE). Vortioxetine had numerically higher remission rates versus all therapies included (ITC). Withdrawal rates due to AEs were significantly lower for vortioxetine versus sertraline, venlafaxine and bupropion, and numerically lower versus citalopram. Switching to vortioxetine was statistically superior to escitalopram in improving treatment emergent sexual dysfunction (TESD). Tolerability was similarly good in the switch and overall MDD populations. These findings suggest vortioxetine is an effective switch therapy for patients with MDD whose response to SSRI/SNRI therapy is inadequate. Vortioxetine was well tolerated and, for patients with a history of TESD, showed significant advantages versus escitalopram. Vortioxetine appears to be a valid option for patients with MDD who have not been effectively treated with first-line pharmacotherapies.[22]

Targeting other Pathways in Treatment-Resistant Depression

In the preceding sections the evidence regarding the currently available psychotherapeutic agents was recapitulated. In this regard, there is a great need for novel agents which can target the pathogenic mechanisms in mood disorders, as lasting cures could only be achieved through this approach. Innovative pathways of emerging importance are the following: the inflammatory pathway, the oxidative and nitrosative stress (O&NS) pathways, the hypothalamic–pituitary–adrenal (HPA) axis, neurotrophic signaling pathway, the metabolic and bioenergetics system, the glutamate system, the opioid and the cholinergic systems. Numerous current conventional antidepressants have been noted to have some effects on these systems. However, of more interest are the agents being presently explored that predominantly aim at one or more of these unique mechanisms, instead of primarily the monoamine system. Monoamines have been the center of psychopharmacology for the past 70 years and have been targeted from several angles with numerous medications, being fully exhausted of their pharmacologic potential. Despite this

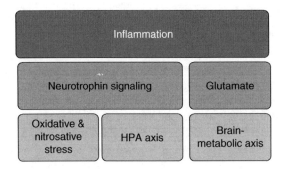

Figure 8.2 Potential targets of novel therapeutic agents in treatment-resistant depression

Major depressive disorder (MDD) is an umbrella term used to describe many dissimilar conditions that have differing pathogenic pathways. This figure illustrates the mechanistic routes with the most evidence of involvement in the etiopathology of MDD. By targeting these mechanisms it is possible to find cures for people with mood disorders in general, and TRD in particular.

fact, mood disorders remain challenging conditions to manage and place an immense burden on the individual and their families. Therefore, the impetus for discovering genuinely novel agents acting outside of the monoamine cascades is compelling. Figure 8.2 schematically depicts the major mechanistic routes that are considered to play a role in TRD, and focusing on these targets holds therapeutic promise.

The Inflammatory Pathway

A possible pathophysiological mechanism associated with TRD is inflammation. Understanding the inflammatory molecular mechanisms of treatment response may provide new strategies for treatment-resistant patients in order to reduce negative outcomes such as suicidal behavior. Targeting specific cytokines that are associated with suicidal behavior such as IL-2, IL-6, IL-8 and TNFα could help prevent suicidality and increased mortality in TRD patients. To extend this argument further, MDD patients with baseline increased IL-6, low high density lipoprotein (HDL) cholesterol, hypertriglyceridemia and hyperglycemia were less likely to achieve remission after two years of treatment than patients without these inflammatory and metabolic dysregulations.[23]

The evidence of inflammatory processes in MDD has been the rationale for studying the COX-2 inhibitor celecoxib as an adjunctive to antidepressant treatment. A recent meta-analysis evaluated four double-blind, placebo-controlled trials (totaling 150 patients) on adjunctive celecoxib for MDD. Patients receiving adjunctive celecoxib showed a better improvement on depressive symptoms (mean difference = 3.26; 95% CI, 1.81–4.71) as well as higher response (OR = 6.49; 95% CI, 2.89–14.55) and remission (OR = 6.58;

95% CI, 2.55–17.00) rates than patients receiving placebo, and was well tolerated.[24]

A proof-of-concept, double-blind RCT studied TNF antagonist infliximab for 60 TRD patients; although the patients on infliximab did not have a greater improvement in depressive symptoms than patients on placebo, patients with increased TNF at baseline responded more than patients without baseline TNF increase. Also, infliximab-treated responders showed a greater decrease in C-reactive protein (CRP) from baseline to endpoint than placebo-treated patients.[25]

In this regard, a notable interest in natural anti-inflammatory agents has developed as well. Omega-3 polyunsaturated fatty acids are dietary fatty acids that cannot be endogenously produced by humans. These exhibit an anti-inflammatory effect by competing with arachidonic acid for COX enzymes thereby decreasing prostaglandin E2 levels and thus decreasing proinflammatory cytokine production. Omega-3 polyunsaturated fatty acids (O3-PUFA) with > 60% eicosapentaenoic acid content have shown the most potential, with several trials and meta-analyses showing a significant antidepressant effect of O3-PUFA as an adjunct to SSRI therapy in MDD.[26] Curcumin, an Asian spice known to have potent anti-inflammatory and antioxidant effects, has also shown promise in preclinical studies; however, RCTs of curcumin in MDD have provided conflicting results so far. Currently no trials have been conducted to evaluate curcumin or O3-PUFA in TRD samples; therefore, their application to this population is still unknown. These agents are particularly appealing because of their benign tolerability and safety profiles.

Tetracycline antibiotics, doxycycline and minocycline, also have potent anti-inflammatory effects and are currently being evaluated for the treatment of MDD. Preclinical data for minocycline indicate that it exerts antidepressant effects through its anti-inflammatory, antioxidant, anti-glutamatergic and neuroprotective properties.[27] Clinical trials are currently underway to investigate minocycline as an adjunctive therapy for MDD and bipolar depression. Doxycycline has also demonstrated promise, as recent preclinical data show improvement of depressive-like behavioral manifestations in inflammatory mouse models.[28] Currently no clinical trials for tetracycline antibiotics for TRD have been reported; however, because of their preclinical effects, these pleiotropic agents are of interest in TRD.

Oxidative and Nitrosative Stress

An inevitable consequence of the proinflammatory state is O&NS both of which are necessary for physiologic cellular functioning when appropriately regulated. Reactive oxygen species (ROS) and reactive nitrogen species are normally produced during cellular respiration and are counterbalanced by antioxidant defenses such as glutathione (an endogenous antioxidant), enzymes (glutathione peroxidase, catalase, superoxide dismutase), melatonin and coenzyme Q10. Free radicals may react with other molecules such as lipids, proteins and DNA causing damage to these macromolecules, potentially leading to cellular dysfunction. Centrally, increased O&NS has been shown to cause neurotoxicity and impair neuroplasticity and neurogenesis. Not surprisingly, increased levels of O&NS has been linked to several psychiatric disorders, including MDD, as shown in a recent meta-analysis.[29] Therefore, the use of antioxidants may present another novel therapeutic target separate from the monoamine pathway.

N-acetylcysteine (NAC) is a glutathione precursor that has multiple potential antidepressant effects through its pleiotropic actions, including decrease in inflammatory cytokines, modulating glutamate, promoting neurogenesis and reducing cellular apoptosis. NAC has been shown to have antioxidant effects in the anterior cingulate cortex in a multicenter RCT of MDD participants treated with adjunctive NAC. Using spectroscopy, higher glutamate-glutamine (Glx) and N-acetyl-aspartate levels were shown in patients treated with NAC, indicative of an antioxidant effect.[30] Further, in a recent RCT (n=252), MDD patients were randomized to placebo or NAC for 12 weeks. At the 12-week endpoint, there was no statistically significant difference in symptoms; however, by week 16, NAC was shown to be superior. The endpoint of the study was 12 weeks, thus making it a negative trial; nevertheless, the delayed effect may suggest a latency of effect or potential blocking mechanism preventing further damage.[31] Further studies are warranted to assess NAC in the TRD population on a more long-term basis.

Targeting Glutamate

The regulation of the glutamate "tripartite" synapse involves presynaptic and postsynaptic neurons and glia. Multiple different receptors regulate glutamate levels as well as the transmission of downstream effects. The following are key targets involved in determining glutamate levels and effects: excitatory amino acid transporters (EAATs), postsynaptic density proteins, alpha-amino-3-hydroxy-5-methyl-4-isoxazolepropionic acid (AMPA) receptors, N-methyl-D-aspartate (NMDA) receptors, kainate (KA) receptors and cognate metabotropic glutamate (mGlu) receptors. Further, modulations of these receptors have been implicated in preclinical models of mood disorders. Therefore, pharmaceutical manipulation of these targets is currently being investigated for TRD.

Of particular interest has been maneuvering of inotropic glutamate receptors, specifically NMDA and AMPA. Current preclinical and clinical evidence suggests decreased activation of NMDA and increased activation of AMPA receptors leads to a salutary mood outcome. In brief, increased AMPA stimulation relative to NMDA stimulation leads to an influx of calcium and sodium, initiating an intracellular cascade ultimately causing an increased BDNF expression and release, thus facilitating improved neuroplasticity and neuronal function. The mammalian target of rapamycin (mTOR) has been implicated as a point of convergence of these intracellular pathways as mTOR has been shown to inhibit 4E-binding protein (4E-BP), which is known to hinder BDNF production. Notably, mTOR has been shown to be down-regulated in MDD patients and a reversal of this phenomenon is associated with antidepressant effects. AMPA stimulation is associated with activation of the mTOR pathway. Taken together, modulation of the glutamate inotropic receptors to increase AMPA stimulation and decrease NMDA stimulation may lead to downstream effects of increased BDNF, improved neuroplasticity and ultimately improved mood and cognition.[32] Exploiting these mechanisms expectedly has immense prospects for the treatment of TRD.

Ketamine is a voltage dependent NMDA antagonist currently used clinically as an anesthetic agent. Interest in ketamine for other purposes, including MDD, has grown enormously in the past decade. In a recent meta-analysis, seven RCTs using an IV infusion and one RCT using intranasal ketamine were assessed for antidepressant effect in MDD and bipolar depression. This drug was associated with higher rates of clinical remission relative to comparator (saline or midazolam) at 24 hours (OR 7.06, NNT = 5), 3 days (OR 3.86, NNT = 6) and 7 days (OR 4.00, NNT = 6), as well as higher rates of clinical response at 24 hours (OR 9.10, NNT = 3), 3 days (OR 6.77, NNT = 3) and 7 days (OR 4.87, NNT = 4). Ketamine was associated with transient psychotomimetic effects; however, no persistent psychosis or affective switches were noted. Therefore, ketamine presented as a potent, fast acting antidepressant for BD and MDD, completely different from conventional antidepressants, which take days to weeks before an initial antidepressant effect is observed.[33] Further, several clinical trials have also shown an effect of ketamine in the setting of TRD. In a RCT, 18 TRD patients were given an IV infusion of either ketamine hydrochloride (0.5 mg/kg) or placebo on two test days, one week apart. Patients receiving ketamine showed significant improvement in depression ratings compared with patients receiving placebo. The effect was noted within 110 minutes after injection and remained significant throughout the following week.[34] Similar results were observed in several other clinical trials; of note, two additional RCTs have shown an anti-suicidal effect of ketamine in the TRD population.[35] A large number of trials of ketamine for TRD are presently underway as interest grows in NMDA modulation; however, the clinical applicability is currently extremely limited due to its short duration of effect. Long-term side effects of ketamine are yet to be assessed. Concern over side effects observed in patients abusing ketamine has prompted concern and stigmatization to the treatment. However, it is important to note that observational data in substance abuse populations should not be directly applied as the dosage varies greatly and it is unclear if these patients are co-administering other drugs of abuse, altering the perceived side effect profile interpreted from this patient group.

One-Carbon Metabolism

The one-carbon cycle is a metabolic pathway that enables the methylation of intracellular molecules. The cycle is required in the synthesis of monoamine neurotransmitters including serotonin, dopamine and norepinephrine.

Therefore, dysfunction of the one-carbon cycle has been investigated as another potential cause of MDD. Of particular interest in MDD has been S-adenosyl-methionine (SAMe) and L-methyl-folate, key naturally occurring compounds involved in the one-carbon cycle. Indeed, decreased levels of folate and SAMe have been linked to MDD. Further, supplementation of folate and SAMe has been shown repeatedly in RCTs to improve MDD symptoms. Mechanistically, supplementation of SAMe and folate provide donor methyl groups thus increasing the synthesis of monoamines. SAMe is also upstream of creatine production and may be partly exerting its antidepressant effects through this bioenergetics pathway. A new trial studied 73 TRD patients in a six-week, double-blind RCT of adjunctive oral SAMe (target dose: 800 mg/twice daily). The HRSD response rate was significantly higher for participants treated with adjunctive SAMe (36.1% v 17.6%) with a NNT of 7.[36] Furthermore, several RCTs and meta-analyses have shown a positive effect of SAMe for MDD.[37] Correspondingly, L-methyl-folate has been shown to increase monoamine levels and improve MDD symptoms in many studies. Of note, important other mechanisms of action have been proposed for SAMe and L-methyl-folate including regulation of oxidative stress as well as anti-inflammatory effects.

Mitochondrial Bioenergetics

Neuronal mitochondrial dysfunction may impair ATP production, promote ROS formation, inappropriately increase intracellular calcium and induce neuronal apoptosis. Mitochondrial dysfunction has been repeatedly linked to MDD and other psychiatric disorders and this organelle's modulators may present novel targets for TRD. Increasing intracellular energy stores would buffer against potential mitochondrial dysfunction which leads to decreased ATP levels. In this regard, decreased levels of creatine monohydrate have been observed in MDD patients. Further, supplementation of creatine leads to a shift in creatine kinase activity with increased production of phosphocreatine (PCr), a high-energy molecule used as intracellular energy. Indeed, preclinical studies with creatine supplementation have been encouraging and lead to antidepressant-like effects and heightened motivation in animal models. In a recently published RCT, 3–5 g of creatine monohydrate was added to escitalopram in 52 females with TRD. After eight weeks of treatment improvement in depressive symptoms was greater in patients receiving creatine augmentation relative to placebo. MDD-related metabolic and network dysfunction as measured by functional neuroimaging also significantly improved in the creatine group, underscoring the fact that positive effects of creatine monohydrate on brain bioenergetics and network organization may partly underlie its efficacy in TRD.[38] Encouraging findings from preliminary investigations have prompted several RCTs which are currently underway, and in this regard the benign side effect profile of creatine supplementation is an appealing factor to allow wider investigation in TRD populations.

The Hypothalamic–Pituitary–Adrenal Axis

Dysregulation of the HPA axis and failure of negative feedback loops has been noted in TRD. The findings in this regard are:

a) Loss of diurnal variation of cortisol.
b) Excessive blood cortisol levels in the evening.
c) Flattening of the cortisol curve with persistent hypercortisolemia.
d) Insensitivity of the glucocorticoid receptor (GR).
e) Increased activity of the GR chaperone protein, FKBP5.

Excess cortisol has been shown to have potent negative effects on mood. Several downstream mechanisms may be at play including the increased activity of indoleamine 2, 3 dioxygenase leading to decreased serotonin and increased levels of TRYCATs (tryptophan catabolites). Therefore, preventing hypercortisolemia may serve as another novel target. Of particular interest has been metyrapone, a cortisol synthesis inhibitor (inhibitor of 11-β hydroxylase, the enzyme that catalyzes the conversion of 11-deoxycortisol to cortisol). Several open-label trials showed a positive effect of metyrapone on TRD. Further, in a RCT with 63 in-patients with severe MDD, augmentation of nefazodone or fluvoxamine for three weeks with placebo versus 1 g of metyrapone once daily was assessed. The metyrapone group showed a significantly greater improvement compared with the placebo group (effect size of 0.6) using response (a decrease in HRSD score by 50%, five weeks post initiation of treatment) as the outcome measure.[39] One additional RCT has been completed; however, results are yet to be published. Oxytocin has also been shown to be a potent suppressor of the HPA axis. Intranasal oxytocin is therefore being currently investigated in a RCT for TRD.

The Neurotrophin Signaling Cascade in Mood Disorders

Neurotrophins are shown to be vital for neurogenesis, neuroplasticity, dendrite formation and synaptogenesis throughout development and in adulthood. A relative decrease in neurotrophins centrally and peripherally has been implicated in the pathogenesis of MDD. Moreover, the decrease in neurotrophin levels in MDD has been implicated in the observed decrease in volume and synaptic connectivity of the prefrontal cortex, amygdala and hippocampus, areas notably involved in mood and cognition. Logically, this decrease in connectivity and volume may lead to less functional neuronal circuits and ultimately poorer emotional and cognitive function, as observed in MDD. Of particular interest in relation to MDD have been BDNF levels. In fact, decreased levels of BDNF appear to be associated with MDD.[40] Further, many of the other pathways (inflammation, oxidative stress, metabolic-brain axis, glutamate system) appear to converge on BDNF signaling. Moreover, several conventional antidepressants have been shown to increase BDNF levels.

More recently, ketamine has been revealed to potently increase BDNF levels and have a strong immediate antidepressant effect in TRD patients, further bolstering the role of this neurotrophin in the pathogenesis of TRD.[41]

Also of interest has been erythropoietin (EPO), an endogenously produced glycoprotein hormone well known for its physiologic effect of increasing erythropoiesis. Erythropoietin is also produced in the brain where it has potent neuroprotective effects mediated through signaling pathways boosting BDNF levels. Centrally, EPO is known to activate anti-apoptotic pathways, promote dendritic sprouting and neurogenesis while also having antioxidant and anti-inflammatory effects. Importantly, systemically administered EPO has been shown to cross the blood–brain barrier and exert the aforementioned downstream effects. Therefore, systemic administration of EPO has been evaluated for its effect on TRD.

In a double-blind, placebo-controlled, parallel-group design, 40 TRD patients were randomized to eight-weekly EPO (40,000 IU) or saline infusions. Patients were assessed at baseline and at weeks 5, 9 and 14 for improvement in depressive symptoms and cognition. HRSD scores and remission rates did not reveal beneficial effects of EPO over saline at week 9; however, EPO improved Beck Depression Inventory (BDI) and World Health Organization Quality Of Life-BREF) (WHO QOL-BREF) scores, and this effect was maintained at follow-up week 14. Moreover, EPO enhanced verbal recall and recognition, which was sustained at follow-up. Although the trial had a negative primary outcome (no HRSD improvement compared to control), improvement in other depression scores and cognitive function provide an impetus for further investigating EPO's therapeutic effects in TRD in larger trials. While the clinical relevance is low for improved depression scores without remission, its potential role in improved cognition for TRD patients is significant.[42]

The Brain-Metabolic Axis

Diabetes, obesity and metabolic syndrome have been shown to have a bidirectional relationship with mood disorders. Plausibly, metabolic dysfunction has several pathways by which brain function may be impaired in the realms of mood and cognition. Preclinical models have shown that insulin resistance may decrease the transport of insulin across the blood–brain barrier leading to decreased central insulin levels. Insulin serves as a potent growth factor in the brain, increasing levels of BDNF and vascular endothelial growth factor, especially having trophic effects on the amygdala, hippocampus and prefrontal cortex, areas essential to the regulation of emotion and cognition. As well, glucose uptake is partly insulin dependent in these brain regions via the Glut4 insulin dependent glucose transporter. Therefore, reduced central insulin levels may lead to diminished intracellular glucose concentrations in key brain areas causing failure in long-term potentiation, decreased neural plasticity and ultimately decline in emotional as well as cognitive functions.

Taken together, poor neuronal function secondary to insulin resistance may serve as a potential cause of TRD as this pathway is minimally affected by monoamine-based therapies. This hypothesis has led to the repurposing of anti-diabetic medications for treatment of MDD.[43] Of particular interest has been the use of incretins, insulin sensitizers and insulin. Currently no clinical trials have been conducted using anti-diabetic medications for the treatment of TRD; however, clinical trials showing the effective use of these medications as an adjunct to conventional antidepressant therapies for MDD provide the impetus for evaluation of their use in TRD, specifically in the large subpopulation of such patients with comorbid metabolic dysfunction. Particularly promising agents include intranasal insulin, glucagon like peptide-1 (GLP-1) analogs and pioglitazone.

Pioglitazone is a thiazolidinedione drug used primarily in the diabetic population as an insulin sensitizer. The primary mechanism of action is through stimulation of peroxisome proliferator-activated receptor gamma (PPARγ). Stimulation of PPARγ has anti-inflammatory, antioxidant and neuroprotective effects, while preclinical studies also suggest modulation of NMDA receptors by pioglitazone. The multiple neuroprotective effects of PPARγ stimulation appears to be mediated through modulation of the parainflammatory and endoplasmic reticulum stress responses.[44] Parainflammation is an inflammatory response to "new" stimuli of the modern era that have not been seen earlier in evolution and therefore appropriate responses have yet to be selected for. Examples of such stimuli include exposure to novel foodstuffs and chemicals, alteration in light–dark exposure patterns, obesity, type 2 diabetes, sedentary lifestyle, atherosclerosis, aging and emotional stress. These stimuli prompt the attempt to restore homeostasis, which leads to chronic activation of acute stress pathways including the stimulation of the innate immune system and subsequent release of proinflammatory cytokines. The PPARγ system when activated prevents the perpetuation of the parainflammatory response and is thus neuroprotective against the deleterious effects of a prolonged inflammatory reaction.

Clinical data in support of pioglitazone's use for MDD has also been accumulating. In a 12-week, open-label, flexible-dose study, 23 patients with MDD received pioglitazone monotherapy or adjunctive therapy initiated at 15 mg daily. Pioglitazone decreased depression symptom severity from a total Inventory of Depressive Symptomatology (IDS) score of 40.3±1.8 to 19.2±1.8 at week 12 ($p<.001$) and a significant reduction in inflammation as measured by log hs-CRP (-0.87±0.72; $p<.001$). Also of note, the majority of participants (74%, n=17) had already failed at least one antidepressant trial.[45] These results were replicated in a double-blind, placebo-controlled RCT with 40 patients with MDD randomized to citalopram plus pioglitazone (15 mg every 12 h) or citalopram plus placebo for six weeks. Pioglitazone showed superiority over placebo during the course of the trial.[46] These results were reproduced in a six-week double-blinded RCT with 50 patients with comorbid polycystic ovarian syndrome and MDD.[47] While there has yet to be a trial specific for TRD, there has been one case report for TRD treated effectively with pioglitazone.[48]

These pathways would be of particular interest in TRD as the brain-metabolic axis is largely unaffected by monoamine agents. Therefore, insulin sensitivity and metabolic dysfunction could represent a subgroup of TRD patients that monoamine therapy would be particularly not useful for. Indeed, in further support of this hypothesis epidemiologic data suggest metabolic dysfunction is a major risk factor of TRD. Of note, these targets are usually extremely well tolerated with mild side effect profiles and well studied in the diabetic population. Limitations of use of these targets largely relate to selecting the subgroup of TRD patients that may benefit, i.e., TRD patients with perfect metabolic function and insulin sensitivity might not benefit from insulin-based therapies.

Conclusion

This chapter summarizes the current conventional pharmacological strategies available for managing TRD. The diversity of treatments reflects the complexity of MDD, in which a single approach cannot account for the varied facets of the disorder. Due to this intricacy, the management of TRD should ideally target the alternate factors relevant to each patient. The paucity of strong evidence to guide clinical decision reflects the need for larger and well-designed studies in TRD. Switching from an SSRI to venlafaxine is a strategy supported by the literature, although the advantage of switching to venlafaxine over other SSRIs is not clear. However, in more severe cases of TRD, venlafaxine was shown to be on the whole useful. The combination of antidepressants, especially mirtazapine, may be beneficial for some patients with TRD, although further studies are needed to establish the superiority of this regimen. Augmentation of antidepressants with lithium or T3 has received wide support in the literature, but in most of the studies they have been evaluated as adjunctive drugs to TCAs and the effect sizes are usually small. AAPs have shown good efficacy as augmentation agents in several well-designed studies and meta-analyses, but metabolic side effects may limit their use. Moreover, the lack of independent trials is a limitation of the studies on AAP. While there are some promising results on the use of modafinil as an augmentation strategy, the role of psychostimulants in TRD is not yet established. Vortioxetine is a promising new antidepressant with effects on core depressive symptoms as well as cognition. Recently, it has been shown to be effective as a switch agent in patients who have failed to respond to an adequate trial of a conventional drug.

The need for novel targets acting outside of the monoamine system is of great importance as rates of TRD are high while using monoamine modulators alone. Several pathogenic pathways may yield novel targets for TRD and many of these are inter-connected. For instance, increased inflammation may lead to increased oxidative stress and overactivity of the HPA axis, which

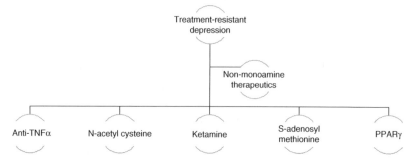

Figure 8.3 Novel therapeutic agents with evidence of efficacy in treatment-resistant depression

Several lines of evidence point to the fact that the depressive phenotype manifests through diverse pathogenic pathways. By only targeting the monoamine neurotransmission, currently available antidepressants show poor efficacy in a large minority of MDD patients. The research community is earnestly trying to unravel the mechanisms that are responsible for treatment non-response. This figure illustrates novel therapeutic agents that have shown efficacy in controlled or well-conducted open-label studies. See text for a detailed account of promising new drugs in treatment-resistant depression.

has modulatory effects on the glutamate system, autonomic nervous system and monoamine neurotransmission. Agents targeting each of these pathways were described here. Of note, several of the alternatives discussed have been shown to affect multiple pathways directly and indirectly. For many of the targets delineated, preclinical data is highly encouraging and informative of potential mechanisms underlying TRD. Clinical data for these agents is still greatly limited as many of the trials discussed were open-label and/or had small numbers of participants. Therefore, the generalized clinical applicability of these agents in TRD remains uncertain. Further, based on current evidence the clinical use of any of the agents described here could not be recommended. Several clinical trials for these medications are currently underway and as such there is still hope for more definitive evidence in the near future in support for or against the contended targets. Figure 8.3 diagrammatically portrays the foremost medications that are of proven value in TRD and act outside of the monoamine neurotransmission.

In using novel targets acting outside of the monoamine pathways, identifying the reason for TRD on an individual basis may allow correction of the cause of the TRD in the specific patient instead of simply using trial and error until an effective agent or combination of agents is found. Therefore, the use of biomarkers to identify the dysfunctional pathway causing nonresponse to conventional therapies may inform the target most likely to have success in a specific TRD patient. This form of treatment selection may also help in designing future clinical trials for TRD to more adequately choose a patient population of interest rather than grouping all cases together, based solely on treatment nonresponse to conventional therapies.

Summary Points

- MDD is likely a constellation of different conditions with varying etiologies and diverging pathogenic pathways.
- The standard antidepressants are all based on the paradigm of monoamine dysregulation.
- Only one-third of MDD patients achieve remission with an initial trial of a conventional antidepressant.
- Therefore, different strategies including switching, combination and augmentation have been tested.
- Nonetheless, approximately one-third of patients remain treatment refractory in spite of multiple drug trials.
- As such, research has been directed towards defining novel pathways which may be implicated in TRD.
- These include the immune-inflammatory pathway, the oxidative stress pathway, the HPA axis, the brain-metabolic axis, the glutamatergic system and the neurotrophin pathway.
- Based on unique targets, new agents have been tested but several caveats have prevented new therapies from entering into clinical usage.
- While there is robust preclinical proof, large well-controlled trials are needed before novel treatments can be applied in clinical practice.

References

1) Trevino K, McClintock SM, McDonald Fischer N, Vora A, Husain MM. Defining treatment-resistant depression: a comprehensive review of the literature. Ann Clin Psychiatry 2014;26:222–232.

2) Peeters FP, Ruhe HG, Wichers M, Abidi L, Kaub K, van der Lande HJ, et al. The Dutch measure for quantification of treatment resistance in depression (DM-TRD): an extension of the Maudsley Staging Method. J Affect Disord 2016;205:365–371.

3) Poirier MF, Boyer P. Venlafaxine and paroxetine in treatment-resistant depression. Double-blind, randomised comparison. Br J Psychiatry 1999;175:12–16.

4) Lenox-Smith AJ, Jiang Q. Venlafaxine extended release versus citalopram in patients with depression unresponsive to a selective serotonin reuptake inhibitor. Int Clin Psychopharmacol 2008;23:113–119.

5) Baldomero EB, Ubago JG, Cercós CL, Ruiloba JV, Calvo CG, López RP. Venlafaxine extended release versus conventional antidepressants in the remission of depressive disorders after previous antidepressant failure: ARGOS study. Depress Anxiety 2005;22:68–76.

6) Nierenberg AA, Papakostas GI, Petersen T, Kelly KE, Iacoviello BM, Worthington JJ, et al. Nortriptyline for treatment-resistant depression. J Clin Psychiatry 2003;64:35–39.

7) Thase ME, Rush AJ, Howland RH, Kornstein SG, Kocsis JH, Gelenberg AJ, et al. Double-blind switch study of imipramine or sertraline treatment of antidepressant-resistant chronic depression. Arch Gen Psychiatry 2002;59:233–239.

8) McGrath PJ, Stewart JW, Fava M, Trivedi MH, Wisniewski SR, Nierenberg AA, et al. Tranylcypromine versus venlafaxine plus mirtazapine following three

failed antidepressant medication trials for depression: a STAR*D report. Am J Psychiatry 2006;163:1531–1541.

9) Fang Y, Yuan C, Xu Y, Chen J, Wu Z, Cao L, et al. A pilot study of the efficacy and safety of paroxetine augmented with risperidone, valproate, buspirone, trazodone, or thyroid hormone in adult Chinese patients with treatment-resistant major depression. J Clin Psychopharmacol 2011;31:638–642.

10) Bobo WV, Chen H, Trivedi MH, Stewart JW, Nierenberg AA, Fava M, et al. Randomized comparison of selective serotonin reuptake inhibitor (escitalopram) monotherapy and antidepressant combination pharmacotherapy for major depressive disorder with melancholic features: a CO-MED report. J Affect Disord 2011;133:467–476.

11) Kato M, Takekita Y, Koshikawa Y, Sakai S, Bandou H, Nishida K, et al. Non response at week 4 as clinically useful indicator for antidepressant combination in major depressive disorder. A sequential RCT. J Psychiatr Res 2017;89:97–104.

12) Rocha FL, Fuzikawa C, Riera R, Hara C. Combination of antidepressants in the treatment of major depressive disorder: a systematic review and meta-analysis. J Clin Psychopharmacol 2012;32:278–281.

13) Rush AJ, Trivedi MH, Stewart JW, Nierenberg AA, Fava M, Kurian BT, et al. Combining medications to enhance depression outcomes (CO-MED): acute and long-term outcomes of a single-blind randomized study. Am J Psychiatry 2011;168:689–701.

14) Thase ME, Youakim JM, Skuban A, Hobart M, Zhang P, McQuade RD, et al. Adjunctive brexpiprazole 1 and 3 mg for patients with major depressive disorder following inadequate response to antidepressants: a phase 3, randomized, double-blind study. J Clin Psychiatry 2015;76:1232–1240.

15) Casey DE, Laubmeier KK, Eudicone JM, Marcus R, Berman RM, Rahman Z, et al. Response and remission rates with adjunctive aripiprazole in patients with major depressive disorder who exhibit minimal or no improvement on antidepressant monotherapy. Int J Clin Pract 2014;68:1301–1308.

16) Nelson JC, Rahman Z, Laubmeier KK, Eudicone JM, McQuade RD, Berman RM, et al. Efficacy of adjunctive aripiprazole in patients with major depressive disorder whose symptoms worsened with antidepressant monotherapy. CNS Spectr 2014;19:528–534.

17) McIntyre A, Gendron A, McIntyre A. Quetiapine adjunctive to selective serotonin reuptake inhibitors or venlafaxine in patients with major depressive disorder, comorbid anxiety, and residual depressive symptoms: a randomized, placebo-controlled pilot study. Depress Anxiety 2007;24:487–494.

18) Brotnick B, El-Khalili N, Banov M, Adson D, Datto C, Raines S, et al. Efficacy and tolerability of extended release quetiapine fumarate (quetiapine XR) monotherapy in major depressive disorder: a placebo-controlled, randomized study. J Affect Disord 2011;128:83–94.

19) Trivedi MH, Thase ME, Osuntokun O, Henley DB, Case M, Watson SB, et al. An integrated analysis of olanzapine/fluoxetine combination in clinical trials of treatment-resistant depression. J Clin Psychiatry 2009;70:387–396.

20) Brunner E, Tohen M, Osuntokun O, Landry J, Thase ME. Efficacy and safety of olanzapine/fluoxetine combination vs fluoxetine monotherapy following successful combination therapy of treatment-resistant major depressive disorder. Neuropsychopharmacology 2014;39:2549–2559.

21) Sanchez C, Asin KE, Artigas F. Vortioxetine, a novel antidepressant with multimodal activity: review of preclinical and clinical data. Pharmacol Ther 2015;145:43–57.

22) Thase ME, Danchenko N, Brignone M, Florea I, Diamand F, Jacobsen PL, et al. Comparative evaluation of vortioxetine as a switch therapy in patients with major depressive disorder. Eur Neuropsychopharmacol 2017;[Epub ahead of print].

23) Vogelzangs N, Beekman AT, van ReedtDortland AK, Schoevers RA, Giltay EJ, de Jonge P, et al. Inflammatory and metabolic dysregulation and the 2-year course of depressive disorders in antidepressant users. Neuropsychopharmacology 2014;39:1624–1634.

24) Na KS, Lee KJ, Lee JS, Cho YS, Jung HY. Efficacy of adjunctive celecoxib treatment for patients with major depressive disorder: a meta-analysis. Prog Neuropsychopharmacol Biol Psychiatry 2014;48:79–85.

25) Raison CL, Rutherford RE, Woolwine BJ, Shuo C, Schettler P, Drake DF, et al. A randomized controlled trial of the tumor necrosis factor antagonist infliximab for treatment-resistant depression: the role of baseline inflammatory biomarkers. JAMA Psychiatry 2013;70:31–41.

26) Mocking RJ, Harmsen I, Assies J, Koeter MW, Ruhé HG, Schene AH. Meta-analysis and meta-regression of omega-3 polyunsaturated fatty acid supplementation for major depressive disorder. Transl Psychiatry 2016;6:e756.

27) Majidi J, Kosari-Nasab M, Salari AA. Developmental minocycline treatment reverses the effects of neonatal immune activation on anxiety- and depression-like behaviors, hippocampal inflammation, and HPA axis activity in adult mice. Brain Res Bull 2016;120:1–13.

28) Mello BS, Monte AS, McIntyre RS, Soczynska JK, Custódio CS, Cordeiro RC, et al. Effects of doxycycline on depressive-like behavior in mice after lipopolysaccharide (LPS) administration. J Psychiatr Res 2013;47:1521–1529.

29) Palta P, Samuel LJ, Miller ER 3rd, Szanton SL. Depression and oxidative stress: results from a meta-analysis of observational studies. Psychosom Med 2014;76:12–19.

30) Das P, Tanious M, Fritz K, Dodd S, Dean OM, Berk M, et al. Metabolite profiles in the anterior cingulate cortex of depressed patients differentiate those taking N-acetyl-cysteine versus placebo. Aust N Z J Psychiatry 2013;47:347–354.

31) Berk M, Dean OM, Cotton SM, Jeavons S, Tanious M, Kohlmann K, et al. The efficacy of adjunctive N-acetylcysteine in major depressive disorder: a double-blind, randomized, placebo-controlled trial. J Clin Psychiatry 2014;75:628–636.

32) Abelaira HM, Réus GZ, Ignácio ZM, Dos Santos MA, de Moura AB, Matos D, et al. Ketamine exhibits different neuroanatomical profile after mammalian target of rapamycin inhibition in the prefrontal cortex: the role of inflammation and oxidative stress. Mol Neurobiol 2016;[Epub ahead of print].

33) McGirr A, Berlim MT, Bond DJ, Fleck MP, Yatham LN, Lam RW. A systematic review and meta-analysis of randomized, double-blind, placebo-controlled trials of ketamine in the rapid treatment of major depressive episodes. Psychol Med 2015;45:693–704.

34) Zarate CA Jr, Singh JB, Carlson PJ, Brutsche NE, Ameli R, Luckenbaugh DA, et al. A randomized trial of an N-methyl-D-aspartate antagonist in treatment-resistant major depression. Arch Gen Psychiatry 2006; 63:856–864.

35) Ballard ED, Ionescu DF, VandeVoort JL, Niciu MJ, Richards EM, Luckenbaugh DA, et al. Improvement in suicidal ideation after ketamine infusion: relationship to reductions in depression and anxiety. J Psychiatr Res 2014;58:161–166.

36) Papakostas GI, Mischoulon D, Shyu I, Alpert JE, Fava M. S-adenosyl methionine (SAMe) augmentation of serotonin reuptake inhibitors for antidepressant nonresponders with major depressive disorder: a double-blind, randomized clinical trial. Am J Psychiatry 2010;167:942–948.

37) Sharma A, Gerbarg P, Bottiglieri T, Massoumi L, Carpenter LL, Lavretsky H, et al. S-Adenosylmethionine (SAMe) for neuropsychiatric disorders: a clinician-oriented review of research. J Clin Psychiatry 2017;78:e656-e667.

38) Yoon S, Kim JE, Hwang J, Kim TS, Kang HJ, Namgung E, et al. Effects of creatine monohydrate augmentation on brain metabolic and network outcome measures in women with major depressive disorder. Biol Psychiatry 2016;80:439–447.

39) Jahn H, Schick M, Kiefer F, Kellner M, Yassouridis A, Wiedemann K. Metyrapone as additive treatment in major depression: a double-blind and placebo-controlled trial. Arch Gen Psychiatry 2004;61:1235–1244.

40) Polyakova M, Stuke K, Schuemberg K, Mueller K, Schoenknecht P, Schroeter ML. BDNF as a biomarker for successful treatment of mood disorders: a systematic & quantitative meta-analysis. J Affect Disord 2015;174:432–440.

41) Allen AP, Naughton M, Dowling J, Walsh A, Ismail F, Shorten G, et al. Serum BDNF as a peripheral biomarker of treatment-resistant depression and the rapid antidepressant response: A comparison of ketamine and ECT. J Affect Disord 2015;186:306–311.

42) Miskowiak KW, Vinberg M, Christensen EM, Bukh JD, Harmer CJ, Ehrenreich H, et al. Recombinant human erythropoietin for treating treatment-resistant depression: a double-blind, randomized, placebo-controlled phase 2 trial. Neuropsychopharmacology 2014;39:1399–1408.

43) Kashani L, Omidvar T, Farazmand B, Modabbernia A, Ramzanzadeh F, Tehraninejad ES, et al. Does pioglitazone improve depression through insulin-sensitization? Results of a randomized double-blind metformin-controlled trial in patients with polycystic ovarian syndrome and comorbid depression. Psychoneuroendocrinology 2013;38:767–776.

44) Gold PW, Licinio J, Pavlatou MG. Pathological parainflammation and endoplasmic reticulum stress in depression: potential translational targets through the CNS insulin, klotho and PPAR-γ systems. Mol Psychiatry 2013;18:154–165.

45) Kemp DE, Ismail-Beigi F, Ganocy SJ, Conroy C, Gao K, Obral S, et al. Use of insulin sensitizers for the treatment of major depressive disorder: a pilot study of pioglitazone for major depression accompanied by abdominal obesity. J Affect Disord 2012;136:1164–1173.

46) Sepanjnia K, Modabbernia A, Ashrafi M, Modabbernia MJ, Akhondzadeh S, et al. Pioglitazone adjunctive therapy for moderate-to- severe major depressive disorder: randomized double-blind placebo-controlled trial. Neuropsychopharmacology 2012;37:2093–2100.

47) Kashani L, Omidvar T, Farazmand B, Modabbernia A, Ramzanzadeh F, Tehraninejad ES, et al. Does pioglitazone improve depression through insulin-sensitization? Results of a randomized double-blind metformin-controlled trial in patients with polycystic ovarian syndrome and comorbid depression. Psychoneuroendocrinology 2013;38:767–776.

48) Kemp DE, Ismail-Beigi F, Calabrese JR. Antidepressant response associated with pioglitazone: support for an overlapping pathophysiology between major depression and metabolic syndrome. Am J Psychiatry 2009;166:619.

9 Depressive Phase of Bipolar Disorder

Treatment Recommendations

Introduction

Bipolar disorder (BD) is likely a collection of heterogeneous conditions and best conceptualized as a spectrum disorder. In the American Psychiatric Association's classification, the Diagnostic and Statistical Manual of Mental Disorders – 5th Edition (DSM-5), four conditions are recognized: BD type I, in which there is the occurrence of at least one manic episode in addition to major depressive episodes (MDEs); BD type II, characterized by, at the minimum, one hypomanic episode in addition to MDEs; cyclothymic disorder (hypomanic episodes as well as depressive episodes which fall short of MDEs); and BD not otherwise specified.[1] In a severe manic or depressive episode the patient may experience psychotic symptoms, and if these are mood incongruent, the differentiation from schizoaffective disorder and schizophrenia can become difficult. The term "rapid cycling" is used when a patient has four or more episodes of either polarity in a 12-month period.

Bipolar spectrum disorders have a high prevalence rate of about 4% in the general population.[2] These are chronic, lifelong conditions with the usual onset in adolescence or early adulthood. The index episode is usually an MDE with melancholic features, and the first manic exacerbation may occur several years later in the trajectory of the illness, resulting in an inopportune delay in the correct diagnosis. There is a very high incidence of co-occurring neuropsychiatric conditions, chief among which are substance use and anxiety spectrum disorders.[3] The prognosis of the disease is worsened by the fact that patients can have recurrent and non-remitting depressive episodes. Additionally, the burden of the disorder is further increased by the frequent association of systemic illnesses such as metabolic diseases, cardiovascular disorders, autoimmune diseases and endocrine disorders. Figure 9.1 schematically depicts these notions and illustrates the pernicious nature of BD.

The course of the disease is virulent in a substantial minority of patients, characterized by such poor prognostic features as rapid cycling, mixed states, treatment resistance and comorbidities. Among affected individuals, the recalcitrant nature of the disease is responsible for the excess morbidity and mortality. The depressive symptoms are often intractable and show poor response to

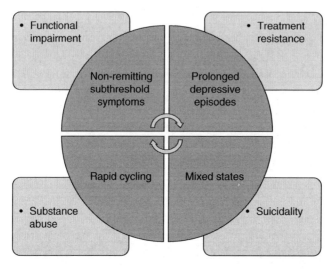

Figure 9.1 The pernicious nature of symptoms in bipolar disorder

In bipolar disorder (BD) many subjects experience self-perpetuating affective disturbances that act in a vicious cycle and lead to such phenomena as rapid cycling, mixed states and persistent subthreshold symptoms. The continued symptomatic state causes myriad complications in the biopsychosocial realm like substance abuse, suicidal tendencies, deterioration of physical health and decline in day-to-day functioning, making BD a very disabling condition.

the currently available psychopharmacological agents.[4] A 15-year prospective follow-up of patients with BD and major depressive disorder (MDD) found depressive, rather than manic, syndromes in the past year were associated with poorer global outcome and greater work disability. Furthermore, recurrent syndromal and sub-syndromal depression was significantly associated with severe overall psychosocial impairment in bipolar, but not unipolar patients.[5]

Antidepressant monotherapy is of little efficacy in bipolar depression and is perhaps contraindicated because of the liability of causing mood destabilization with a switch into mania or hypomania, induction of mixed episodes and rapid cycling. Therefore, the treatment of all phases of BD is primarily with mood stabilizers, which includes first-line agents such as lithium, sodium valproate and carbamazepine. However, the armamentarium has increased in this regard as newer anticonvulsants and atypical antipsychotics are being increasingly employed in the treatment of BD.[6] In addition to mood stabilizing medications, bipolar depression is often responsive to chronotropic interventions, such as single or repeated total sleep deprivation and light therapy. Figure 9.2 gives an overview of the present understanding of the biological treatment of bipolar depression.

The purpose of this chapter is to provide an outline of the pharmacological agents used in the treatment of bipolar depression for which evidence exists in the form of randomized controlled trials (RCTs), and open-label or observational studies. Only those medications that have proven efficacy are

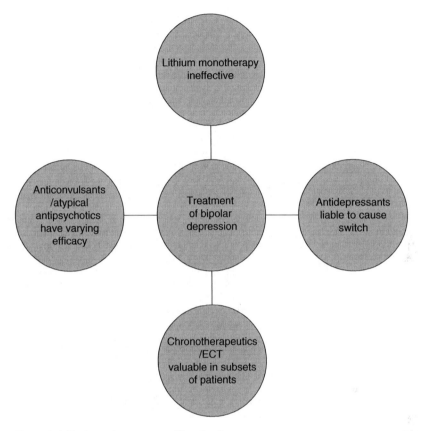

Figure 9.2 Biological treatment of bipolar depression

Bipolar depression is difficult to treat with refractoriness to conventional mood stabilizers like lithium. Used alone, standard antidepressants can cause mood destabilization with switches into manic or hypomanic episodes, induction of mixed states and rapid cycling. Newer anticonvulsants and atypical antipsychotics have varying efficacy in sub-populations of patients with bipolar depression. Chronotherapeutic measures like bright light therapy and total sleep deprivation have good efficacy which is comparable to first-line psychotherapeutic agents. Finally, in treatment refractory cases electroconvulsive therapy is a viable option.

considered, with emphasis on anticonvulsants and atypical antipsychotics, as these are the principal medications employed in the management of this difficult to treat condition.

Lithium and Anticonvulsants

Pharmacodynamic Considerations

Lithium—the prototype mood stabilizer—works, in part, by inhibiting brain glycogen synthase kinase-3 beta (GSK-3β), which is a serine-threonine kinase. GSK-3β is an important member of the human kinome and phosphorylates many transcription factors including nuclear factor-kappa B (NF-κB), heat shock protein factor-1, activator protein-1 and β-catenin, triggering growth factor cascades. Thus, GSK-3β modulates metabolism and survival, the neuronal cytoskeleton and programmed cell death or apoptosis. Enhanced apoptosis is particularly relevant to the induction of manic symptoms in BD, as demonstrated in transgenic murine models in which the experimental animals showed increased manic-like behaviors in line with augmented GSK-3β activity. By downregulating GSK-3β, lithium reduces neuronal apoptosis and leads to the amelioration of manic behaviors.[7]

GSK-3β control is also involved in Wnt signaling pathways that regulate development and cell proliferation. Wnt binds to Frizzled receptors present on cellular membranes and subsequently stimulates a phosphoprotein, the Dishevelled partner DVL-1, which modulates gene expression through β-catenin. This pathway can inactivate GSK-3β and lead to normalization of abnormal behaviors, such as increased talking and social withdrawal, seen in different mood states in BD.[8] It has been demonstrated that both lithium and anticonvulsant mood stabilizers, like sodium valproate and carbamazepine, regulate GSK-3β either by direct inhibition or modulation of downstream effectors. Additionally, anticonvulsants act through further mechanisms such as inhibition of histone deacetylase at the level of the epigenome, and modulation of astrocyte-associated proteins to promote neurogenesis and enhanced connectivity in crucial limbic structures linked to mood regulation.[9] Figure 9.3 gives an illustration of the main pathways through which mood stabilizing medications exert their actions. Table 9.1 provides a selection of studies, giving a representation of the therapeutic impact of the agents described in this section.

Lithium Salts

A literature search revealed only one placebo-controlled, randomized trial of lithium monotherapy in acute BD type I depression that has been published in the last 10 years—the EMBOLDEN I study. In this trial, patients were treated with either quetiapine 300 or 600 mg/d, lithium 600 to 1800 mg/d according to serum levels, or placebo. The duration of the study was eight weeks and the primary outcome measure was change in Montgomery-Asberg Depression Rating Scale (MADRS) from baseline. The results showed that quetiapine (both doses) was significantly more effective than placebo in reducing MADRS total scores but lithium did not reach statistical significance. Additionally, quetiapine was statistically superior to lithium in treating acute bipolar depression, and both treatments were equally well tolerated in the short term.[10] In this scenario, there is a need for further controlled lithium studies to better delineate its place in the management of depressive episodes in BD. Two such trials are ongoing—the ARIQUELI study (efficacy and safety of the combination of aripiprazole or lithium in bipolar patients who are refractory to quetiapine monotherapy) and the comparison of lithium and placebo in suicidal patients in

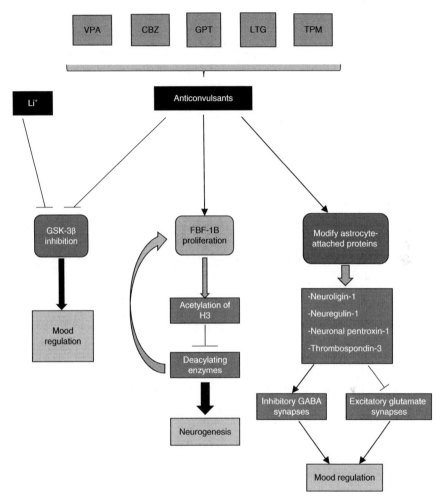

Figure 9.3   The distributed action of lithium ions and anticonvulsants in the regulation of mood

Anticonvulsant mood stabilizers have a pharmacodynamic advantage over lithium in normalizing abnormal manifestations of mood in bipolar disorder. Much like lithium, these modulate the enzyme GSK-3β and its downstream effectors, but additionally the latter act through fibroblast growth factors, histone deacetylation (epigenetic regulation) and astrocyte-attached proteins to stabilize mood.

CBZ – carbamazepine; FBF-1B – fibroblast growth factor-1B; GSK-3β – glycogen synthase kinase-3 beta; GPT – gabapentin; Li⁺ – lithium; LTG – lamotrigine; TPM – topiramate; VPA – valproic acid

affective disorders.[11,12] In conclusion, it can be stated that the current evidence regarding acute bipolar depression is not supportive of lithium monotherapy, but as it is a recalcitrant condition with a substantial suicide risk, adjunctive treatment with this agent may be of value in refractory cases.

Table 9.1 Lithium and anticonvulsants in the treatment of bipolar depression

Medication	Type of research evidence	Findings	Study
Li	RCT	Li compared to PLB and quetiapine. Li did not differ significantly from PLB and was inferior to quetiapine. Conclusion: Li not an effective therapy in acute bipolar depression.	Young et al. (2010)[10]
CBZ	RCT	CBZ (IR) and (XR) compared in BD patients with MADRS and YMRS scores ≥ 15. Both agents equally effective. Conclusion: CBZ effective in both mania and depression.	El-Mallakh et al. (2010)[13]
OXC	RCT	Study population: BD type I and II patients partially responsive to Li therapy. OXC and CBZ added adjunctively and patients followed for eight weeks. Adjunctive OXC significantly more effective than CBZ on efficacy measures. Conclusion: OXC a potentially useful therapy in BD.	Juruena et al. (2009)[14]
ESC	RCT	ESC compared to PLB (three-week trial) in bipolar type I patients with manic episodes. ESC no better than PLB on primary efficacy measure (YMRS). In the continuation phase, ESC showed global reduction in affective symptomatology with good safety profile. Conclusion: ESC may have a place in preventing mood episodes in BD.	Grunze et al. (2015)[15]
DV	Meta-analysis of RCTs	Four RCTs with a total sample size of 142 patients. DV significantly superior to PLB in response and remission rates. Conclusion: DV an effective therapy in acute bipolar depression.	Bond et al. (2010)[18]
LTG	Post hoc analysis	Combined analysis of five RCTs of LTG monotherapy versus PLB in acute bipolar depression. In all trials LTG failed to separate from PLB on main efficacy parameters. Conclusion: LTG no better than PLB in acute bipolar depression.	Calabrese et al. (2008)[19]
TPM	Open-label study	Study sample: BD type I and II patients with refractory mood symptoms and obesity. Open-label TPM added adjunctively and patients studied for 12 weeks. Primary efficacy measure: CGI, secondary parameters: HRSD-21 and YMRS. Patients showed significant improvement on all efficacy measures with a reduction of two points in the body mass index. Conclusion: TPM effective in reducing the severity of mood symptoms and results in significant weight loss.	Gabriel et al. (2007)[36]

GBP	Open-label study	Cases receiving first-line mood stabilizers with therapeutic plasma levels or atypical antipsychotics, but with persistent depressive symptoms, were included (HRSD-28 scores ≥ 18). Open adjunctive GBP added (mean dose 1725 mg/d) and patients followed up for 12 weeks. Those with mild to moderate depression had significant improvement, while the majority of severely depressed subjects did not respond. Conclusion: adjunctive GBP an efficacious therapy in mild to moderate bipolar depression.	Wang et al. (2002)[37]
PGB	Open-label observational study	PGB studied in acute and maintenance periods (2 and 48 months). Subjects: BD spectrum outpatients with treatment resistance. Adjunctive PGB given and bipolar psychopathology measured with CGI-BP. In both parts, significant decrease in symptomatic burden with a prophylactic effect. PGB well tolerated with no serious drug interactions. Conclusion: in BD, PGB is a safe and effective therapy for acute and recurrent mood episodes.	Schaffer et al. (2013)[21]
LVT	RCT	A six-week trial of adjunctive LVT compared to PLB in BD type I or II patients experiencing acute depressive episode. Primary efficacy measure: HRSD-21. Secondary assessments: MADRS, Beck Depression Inventory, Hamilton Anxiety Rating Scale, CGI-BP, and YMRS. With Last Observation Carried Forward, LVT no better than PLB. Conclusion: adjunctive LVT not efficacious in acute bipolar depression.	Saricicek et al. (2011)[23]

BD – bipolar disorder; CBZ – carbamazepine; CGI – clinical global impressions scale; CGI-BP – clinical global impressions scale-bipolar version; DV – divalproex sodium; ESC – eslicarbazepine; GBP – gabapentin; HRSD – Hamilton rating scale for depression; Li – lithium; LTG – lamotrigine; LVT – levetiracetam; MADRS – Montgomery-Asberg depression rating scale; OXC – oxcarbazepine; PGB – pregabalin; PLB – placebo; TPM – topiramate; YMRS – Young Mania Rating Scale

Carbamazepine/Oxcarbazepine/Eslicarbazepine

During the last 10 years no placebo-controlled studies of carbamazepine (CBZ), per se, were found in the extant literature but other work has shed light on its role in BD. Importantly, an investigation compared the efficacy and tolerability of immediate-release (IR) and extended-release (ER) CBZ in BD subjects with acute manic, mixed or depressive episodes. Both BD type I and type II cases were included in the analysis, provided they had MADRS and Young Mania Rating Scale (YMRS) scores ≥15. The patients were already taking CBZ or were considered to benefit from this medication; a comparison of the IR and ER formulations was conducted in a double-blind fashion for the entire study duration of three months. There was a statistically significant decrease in the scores of the efficacy measures with both IR and ER carbamazepine. However, the two compositions did not show any significant difference in their respective outcomes and demonstrated similar adverse effect profiles.[13]

Oxcarbazepine (OXC) is the keto derivative of CBZ. A controlled study of bipolar subjects on lithium monotherapy but with residual symptoms illuminated its role in BD. Conducted in outpatients, cases with an inadequate response to lithium were randomly assigned to either adjunctive CBZ or OXC in a double-blind manner. Fifty-two cases with lingering manic, mixed or depressive symptoms as identified by using SADS-L (Schedule for Affective Disorders and Schizophrenia-Lifetime Version) were selected and followed up for eight weeks. Outcome measures included Hamilton Rating Scale for Depression (HRSD)-21, MADRS, YMRS, Clinical Global Impression-Severity (CGI-S) and Clinical Global Impression-Improvement (CGI-I). All subjects completed the study and results were reported for the observed cases. Both CBZ and OXC were statistically significant in producing improvements on the efficacy measures, but OXC showed greater reductions in a range of affective symptoms than CBZ. Additionally, OXC was associated with fewer adverse events and was better tolerated than CBZ. Thus, while there is still a need for adequately powered studies, this preliminary investigation was useful in showing the utility of OXC in BD.[14]

Eslicarbazepine (ESC), the active enantiomer of metabolized OXC, shares the dibenzazepine ring with its parent compound and CBZ. The drug was approved for epilepsy by the European Medicines Agency in 2009, and since then has been investigated in BD. Presently, it has no approved psychiatric indications, and in a recently published RCT in acute mania, the drug failed to differ from placebo. However, ESC showed valid efficacy on certain outcome measures, in particular the Clinical Global Impression Scale-Bipolar Version (CGI-BP) in the long term.[15] While there are ongoing trials, the verdict is still out on the efficacy of this agent in BD.

Divalproex Sodium

The anticonvulsant, divalproex sodium (DV), is relatively well studied in adults with acute bipolar depression. In a small preliminary study, nine cases with acute non-refractory bipolar depression were compared with nine control subjects for the trial duration of six weeks. The magnitude of reduction in MADRS scores, the primary efficacy measure, was much greater in the treatment arm. Furthermore, a decrease was also observed in YMRS scores, underscoring the efficacy of DV in mixed states.[16]

In a placebo-controlled RCT, patients with BD type I or II, experiencing MDEs and not already on a mood stabilizer, were randomly assigned to divalproex extended-release, or placebo, in a double-blind style. The primary efficacy measure was MADRS and the study duration was six weeks. Sixty-seven percent of the subjects met criteria for rapid cycling; statistical evaluation of the entire study population showed that the active compound was significantly better than placebo in inducing response and remission. Subgroup analysis revealed that in BD type II cases, the drug was not significantly different in outcome from placebo, indicating DV may be more appropriate in acute BD type I depression, particularly in rapid cycling patients. In this short-term study, the drug was associated with gastrointestinal side effects including nausea, increased appetite and diarrhea.[17] In a meta-analysis of four RCTs in acute bipolar depression in adults, DV was found to be superior to placebo with a higher remission rate of 39.3% versus 17.5%.[18]

Lamotrigine

Lamotrigine (LTG) is approved by the United States Food and Drug Administration (FDA) for the maintenance treatment of BD and, in this regard, it may have greater value in preventing depressive relapses than manic relapses. With respect to the treatment of acute bipolar depression, data from controlled trials are not supportive of LTG's efficacy in this group of patients. A study combined the results of five RCTs in acute bipolar depression, comparing LTG monotherapy with placebo. These trials lasted from 7–10 weeks and the active agent was administered at various doses within the therapeutic range. Three studies used a fixed dose of 200 mg/d. In another study, titration was employed, and subsequently the subjects were given a standard dose of either 50 or 200 mg of LTG per day. In the final study, LTG was flexibly dosed from 100–400 mg daily. HRSD-17 was the primary efficacy measure in two of these trials, while MADRS was employed in the remaining studies. In all five studies, LTG failed to show a significantly different outcome from placebo on the main indicators and in only one trial did it show statistical significance on secondary measures such as CGI-S and CGI-I. Nonetheless, the drug was well tolerated in these acute phase studies. In summary, LTG did not show efficacy in the treatment of acute bipolar depression under controlled conditions.[19]

Topiramate

A novel antiepileptic used to treat seizures in patients of all age groups, topiramate (TPM) has been studied in BD, particularly in the treatment of acute episodes. Data from RCTs are available in manic and mixed episodes but no placebo-controlled studies for bipolar depression were identified during the literature search. The following conclusions were drawn from the appraisal of the extant literature.[20] (1) In controlled trials, there is lack of evidence for TPM's efficacy in acute affective episodes. (2) In studies utilizing TPM as an adjunctive agent with primary mood stabilizers and atypical antipsychotics, the drug was well tolerated and no unexpected adverse effects were noted.(3) All studies consistently showed a statistically notable reduction in body mass index. (4) TPM could be employed as an add-on agent in therapy with drugs such as olanzapine, which have a high liability of deranging metabolic parameters, perhaps with additional salutary effects on affective symptomatology. (5) It is FDA approved for the prophylactic treatment of migraine, and may be safely used in people with BD with this comorbidity.

Gabapentin/Pregabalin/Gabapentin Enacarbil

These gamma-aminobutyric acid analogs have the common mechanism of action of binding to the α2δ subunit of voltage-gated calcium channels of presynaptic neurons, decreasing the release of excitatory neurotransmitters and pain mediators. Developed as antiepileptic medications, these are extensively used in the treatment of neuropathic pain of various etiologies. BD psychopathology can be considered as comprising of core affective symptoms and attendant neuropsychiatric manifestations, which are invariable concomitants in the majority of patients. Comorbid anxiety worsens the prognosis because of such factors as persistence of symptoms, mixed episodes, substance misuse and increased suicidality. As such, newer anticonvulsants, including gabapentinoids, are being investigated in bipolar spectrum disorders to provide fresh perspective in a difficult to treat condition. Data from controlled trials are not supportive of the anti-manic efficacy of these compounds, and there is a lack of RCTs in acute bipolar depression. There is some information in the form of case reports, observational studies and prospective trials that show the usefulness of these compounds in acute, as well as maintenance, treatment of BD.[21] In summary, gabapentinoids may have value as adjuncts to first-line mood stabilizers in refractory patients, and patients with anxiety spectrum and substance use disorders as comorbidities. Additionally, these agents may be used in bipolar patients with associated neurological conditions like migraine, neuropathic pain and restless legs syndrome.[22]

Levetiracetam

Levetiracetam (LVT) is a broad spectrum antiepileptic used to treat partial epilepsy, with or without secondary generalization, in children, as well as adults. It has a novel mechanism of action, exerting its effects by binding to the SV2A synaptic vesicle glycoprotein, inhibiting the P/Q type presynaptic calcium channels through an intracellular pathway and resulting in the suppression of glutamate transmission. It has been investigated in BD during acute affective exacerbations, and in treatment refractory patients mostly as an adjunctive agent. While there is evidence of efficacy in subjects experiencing manic, mixed and depressive episodes in non-randomized and open-label trials, this has not been confirmed in RCTs. A single published RCT in acute depression in BD type I and II subjects was conducted with a trial duration of six weeks. The primary efficacy measure was HRSD-21 and secondary evaluation was through MADRS, CGI-BP, Beck Depression Inventory (BDI), Hamilton Anxiety Rating Scale (HAM-A) and YMRS. Forty-two cases were randomly assigned to the active agent or placebo; LVT was flexibly administered and the mean dose was 1132 mg/d at endpoint, with the results reported using the Last Observation Carried Forward (LOCF) method. At endpoint, adjunctive LVT was no better than placebo on primary and secondary outcomes. Under controlled circumstances, add-on LVT was ineffective in treating adult patients with acute bipolar depression.[23]

Atypical Antipsychotics

Pharmacodynamic Considerations

Atypical antipsychotics are a heterogeneous class of medications, having diverse molecular structures but sharing basic mechanisms, which bring about their therapeutic effects. At the dopamine D2 receptor (D2R) level, these medications can be divided into full antagonists, inverse agonists or partial agonists. Risperidone is an example of a full D2R antagonist, olanzapine an inverse agonist and aripiprazole a partial agonist. Murine models of psychosis suggest some of these agents act as functionally selective ligands at the D2R, which is a G-protein coupled receptor (GPCR). Downstream signaling occurs through the adenylyl cyclase-cAMP-PKA cascade, and all antipsychotics activate this pathway. However, novel agents like aripiprazole, brexpiprazole and cariprazine have been shown to selectively work through β-arrestin 2-Akt-GSK-3 signaling at the GPCR which serves as an alternate downstream pathway with ligand binding at the D2R. β-arrestin 2 is a scaffolding protein which activates protein kinase B (Akt), phosphorylating the enzyme GSK-3β, and ultimately causing gene transcription via β-catenin. This cascade appears to control many crucial neuronal functions including expression of receptors and ion conduits, as well as regulation of the process of apoptosis.[24] In affective disorders, there are important implications as critical mood regulating areas in the limbic and paralimbic regions are influenced by this signaling. Figure 9.4 schematically illustrates these concepts. Table 9.2 provides a summation of representative studies of atypical antipsychotics in the treatment of depressive symptoms in BD and related conditions.

Risperidone

Risperidone has been well studied in BD, with evidence of efficacy in manic and mixed episodes in BD type I demonstrated in RCTs. No studies of risperidone as mono or adjunctive therapy in acute bipolar depression were found;

Table 9.2 Second and third generation antipsychotics in the treatment of bipolar depression

Medication	Type of study	Findings	Study
RLAI	Open-label study	Subjects: persistently symptomatic BD patients with rapid cycling while on continuing treatment. Adjunctive RLAI given every two weeks (25–50 mg) for 16 weeks and change in symptomatology measured with CGI-BP-S, YMRS, and MADRS. Significant improvement in affective symptomatology at endpoint, Last Observation Carried Forward. Conclusion: RLAI effective and safe therapy in treatment refractory bipolar patients.	Macfadden et al. (2011)[25]
PDP	RCT	PDP monthly mono or adjunctive therapy in a 15-month relapse prevention trial in schizoaffective disorder. Diagnosis with Structured Clinical Interview for DSM-5 axis I disorders; primary endpoint – time to any relapse: psychotic, manic or depressive. Monthly PDP intramuscular superior to PLB in decreasing active mood or psychotic symptoms and improved functioning. Conclusion: PDP effective in reducing global psychopathology and well tolerated.	Fu et al. (2015)[26]
OZP	Post hoc analysis	Pooled analysis of two monotherapy trials in BD type I depression. Data stratified with respect to MADRS total, MADRS-6 and individual item scores (suicidal patients excluded). OZP significantly superior to PLB on all parameters at week 6. Conclusion: OZP an efficacious therapy for acute depressive episodes in BD type I.	Tohen et al. (2013)[27]
OFC	RCT	Patients with acute bipolar type I depression (MADRS ≥ 20) randomized to OZP, OFC or PLB. Primary efficacy measure: change in MADRS score at endpoint (week 8). Both OZP and OFC significantly superior to PLB; OFC statistically better than OZP with higher remission rates. OFC did not cause manic/hypomanic switch. Conclusion: OFC more effective than OZP in the treatment of acute bipolar type I depression.	Tohen et al. (2003)[28]
QTP	Meta-analysis of RCTs	Eleven short-term trials included. Majority compared QTP monotherapy with placebo. Participants had either BD type I or II. Primary efficacy measure was change from MADRS score at baseline. As monotherapy, QTP showed difference from PLB from week 1 and statistically meaningful difference maintained until endpoint. Conclusion: QTP an effective and well-tolerated treatment in acute bipolar depression in adults.	Suttajit et al. (2014)[29]

ZRD	Post hoc analysis	ZRD monotherapy compared to PLB in two acute six-week trials. Patients (Hamilton Rating Scale for Depression-17 scores ≥ 20) randomized to PLB or ZRD (fixed-flexibly dosed from 40 to 160 mg/d). Primary outcome – MADRS; mixed-model repeated-measure analysis. In both studies ZRD failed to differ from PLB on the primary efficacy measure. Conclusion: ZRD no better than PLB in acute bipolar type I depression.	Lombardo et al. (2012)[30]
LRD	RCT	Cases with bipolar type I depression randomized to LRD (20–60 mg/d), LRD (80–120 mg/d) or PLB. Subjects followed for six weeks, efficacy assessed with MADRS (primary) and CGI-BP (secondary). LRD (either dose) superior to PLB on both outcomes. LRD therapy associated with minimal metabolic side effects. Conclusion: LRD monotherapy safe and effective for acute bipolar I depression.	Loebel et al. (2014)[32]
APZ	RCT	APZ monotherapy versus PLB in outpatients with nonpsychotic, non-suicidal acute bipolar type I depression. AZP flexibly dosed from 5–30 mg/d. Assessments: MADRS (primary outcome) and CGI-BP-S (main secondary outcome). At study conclusion (week 8) APZ failed to differ from PLB. Conclusion: APZ not an efficacious treatment for acute bipolar I depression.	Thase et al. (2008)[34]
CPZ	RCT	Cases with acute bipolar type I depression randomized to PLB or CPZ 0.75, 1.5 or 3 mg/d. All four groups assessed with MADRS (primary) and CGI-BP-S (secondary). Analysis with mixed-model, repeated-measures methodology on the modified intent-to-treat population. Only CPZ 1.5 mg/d achieved statistical significance at endpoint (week 6). CPZ well tolerated with no serious safety concerns. Conclusion: CPZ 1.5 mg/d an efficacious and safe treatment for acute bipolar I depression.	Durgam et al. (2015)[35]

APZ – aripiprazole; BD – bipolar disorder; CGI-BP – clinical global impressions scale – bipolar version; CGI-BP-S – clinical global impressions scale – bipolar-severity of illness scale; CPZ – cariprazine; LRD – lurasidone; MADRS – Montgomery-Asberg depression rating scale; OZP – olanzapine; OFC – olanzapine/fluoxetine combination; PDP – paliperidone palmitate; PLB –placebo; QTP – quetiapine; RCT – randomized controlled trial; RLAI – risperidone long-acting injectable; YMRS – Young Mania Rating Scale; ZRD -ziprasidone

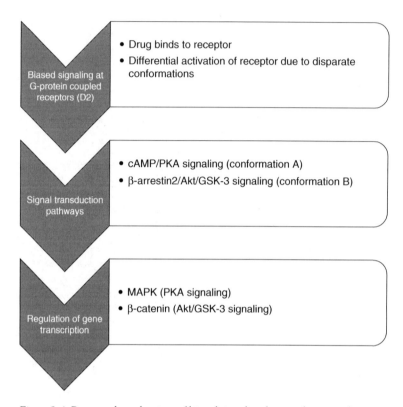

Figure 9.4 Purported mechanism of biased signaling by novel antipsychotics

Biased ligands are presumed to act in a functionally discriminating manner at G-protein coupled receptors, e.g., D2-type dopamine receptors. One method of functional selectivity may be the favored binding to diverse conformations of the receptors, activating different downstream pathways according to the local environment and the neuronal subtypes in which these are expressed. Postsynaptic scaffolding proteins, adaptors and effectors may be affected variably by each receptor conformation related cascade, differentially stimulated by the ligand.

Akt – protein kinase B; cAMP – cyclic adenosine monophosphate; GSK-3 – glycogen synthase kinase-3; MAPK – mitogen activated protein kinase; PKA – protein kinase A

nonetheless, the value of this drug in the treatment of core affective symptoms was shown in a recently published study. The investigators used risperidone long-acting injection (RLAI) in symptomatic BD patients with rapid cycling. In this open-label trial, subjects were marked as having acute depressive or manic/mixed episodes according to their scores on MADRS and YMRS. Cases with MADRS scores ≥16 were considered as having depressive episodes, while those with YMRS scores ≥16 and any MADRS score were deemed as having manic or mixed episodes. RLAI was given intramuscularly in a dose of 25–50 mg every two weeks for the study period of 16 weeks. Statistical examination showed there was significant improvement in CGI-BP and MADRS in depressed subjects, while those with manic and mixed symptoms had notable improvement on YMRS. This analysis called for prospective controlled trials of RLAI in BD subjects with acute exacerbations of any polarity.[25]

Paliperidone or 9-hydroxyrisperidone, the principal metabolite of risperidone, is FDA approved for the treatment of schizophrenia and schizoaffective disorder. In a recently published trial, paliperidone palmitate has shown efficacy in the prevention of psychotic, depressive and manic symptoms in schizoaffective disorder, but further studies are required to prove its efficacy in BD.[26]

Olanzapine

Olanzapine, a second generation antipsychotic (SGA), has been studied in acute phases of BD. The drug is FDA approved as monotherapy for manic and mixed episodes of BD type I, and its efficacy has also been shown in acute bipolar depression in adults. A post hoc analysis of two RCTs demonstrated olanzapine's effectiveness in acute MDEs in BD type I. Olanzapine was employed as monotherapy in a six-week placebo-controlled trial; 690 patients were randomized to the active agent and 524 to placebo. Data of the study subjects were stratified according to change from baseline in MADRS total score, MADRS-6 sub-score and individual item scores. Further, demographic and disease characteristics such as psychotic features, melancholic characteristics and mixed symptoms (defined as scoring ≥ 2 in ≥ 3 YMRS items) were also categorized. Analysis of variance with multiple regression analysis showed that, compared to placebo, the olanzapine group had statistically significant score reductions on all efficacy measures except two MADRS items, namely concentration difficulties and suicidal thoughts. The disease factor that best corresponded to better treatment outcome with olanzapine was the presence of melancholic features in the presentation at the start of the study. In summary, olanzapine monotherapy improved key depressive symptoms in BD type I.[27] In addition, olanzapine in combination with fluoxetine is FDA approved for the treatment of acute bipolar depression in adults.[28]

Quetiapine

This atypical antipsychotic is extensively studied in all phases of BD; it is FDA approved for the treatment of manic and mixed episodes of BD type I, and is also licensed as monotherapy for acute bipolar depression. In addition, it is endorsed as a maintenance agent for the prevention of affective episodes, as an adjunct to mood stabilizers. A systematic review and meta-analysis was conducted of RCTs of quetiapine in acute bipolar depression, providing an estimation of its efficacy and safety. The authors conducted an extensive search of different databases including MEDLINE, CINAHL, PsychINFO, etc., leading to the identification of 11 RCTs. The total number of participants was 3488 with either BD type I or II. Quetiapine was used as monotherapy in the majority of the trials, and compared to placebo or other treatments, such as lithium and selective serotonin reuptake inhibitors (SSRIs). The primary efficacy measure was change in MADRS scores from baseline to the end of study period. Secondary assessments included CGI-BP-S, CGI-S, HAM-A, Sheehan Disability Scale, Pittsburgh Sleep Quality Index, and Quality of Life and Enjoyment and Satisfaction Questionnaire-Short Form. Quetiapine was significantly more effective than placebo on mean reductions in MADRS total scores, and differences in this regard were observed as early as week 1. Furthermore, the active agent was also superior on all secondary efficacy measures. In comparison to the other treatments, quetiapine was better than lithium and paroxetine (EMBOLDEN I and II studies) on the chief outcome parameter. In conclusion, quetiapine was an efficacious treatment for acute bipolar depression with a good safety and tolerability profile.[29]

Ziprasidone

Ziprasidone, an SGA, has been studied as mono or adjunctive therapy in BD, and is FDA licensed for the treatment of manic and mixed episodes. Two RCTs were conducted comparing ziprasidone alone with placebo in patients with MDEs associated with BD. A cut-off score of 20 was used for HRSD-17 to identify BD patients with MDE and cases were randomized to ziprasidone 40 to 160 mg/d or placebo and followed for six weeks. The principal efficacy parameter was change in MADRS scores at baseline, while secondary measures included HRSD and CGI-I. In both studies, the active agent did not differ significantly from placebo on the main assessment measure.

Additionally, in another RCT in acute bipolar depression, ziprasidone in combination with a mood stabilizer (lithium, valproate or lamotrigine) was compared with placebo and mood stabilizer. In this trial too, adjunctive ziprasidone was no better than mood stabilizer alone in patients with bipolar depression.[31] These data suggest ziprasidone does not have efficacy in bipolar depression in controlled situations.

Lurasidone

Lurasidone, another SGA, is unique in that it has FDA approval for the treatment of MDE in BD type I, but so far is not licensed for use in manic or mixed episodes. This endorsement is based on two pivotal internationally conducted RCTs in which lurasidone showed superiority over placebo both as monotherapy and as an adjunct to lithium and valproate. Trial duration was six weeks; patients had acute bipolar depression without psychotic features as determined by the Mini-International Neuropsychiatric Interview and were treated as outpatients. The primary efficacy measure was reduction in total MADRS score at baseline and key secondary assessment was with the CGI-BP depression severity sub-score. In these trials, lurasidone (flexibly dosed from 20–120 mg/d) was superior to placebo on both parameters, showed a good safety profile and was not associated with significant extrapyramidal or metabolic side effects.[32,33] While there is a need for corroborating independent studies, lurasidone does emerge as an important medication for the treatment of acute bipolar depression.

Aripiprazole

Aripiprazole is also referred to as a "third generation antipsychotic" and shows the pharmacodynamic characteristics of partial agonism, functional selectivity and serotonin-dopamine activity modulation. It is well studied in different phases of BD and is FDA licensed for manic and mixed episodes of BD type I as monotherapy, and as maintenance treatment in conjunction with a mood stabilizer. Two RCTs of aripiprazole (flexibly dosed from 5–30 mg/d) were conducted in bipolar depression as standalone therapy in comparison to placebo. These were multicenter, eight-week trials of outpatients with nonpsychotic bipolar I depression; the studies were well-powered and utilized change in MADRS total score as the primary outcome measure. CGI-BP depression severity sub-score was the chief secondary assessment parameter; LOCF was used to account for drop-outs. The active agent showed an early difference from placebo treatment, but at week 8 failed to demonstrate statistically significant superiority on both key primary and secondary efficacy measures. Aripiprazole was less well tolerated than placebo, with a higher incidence of akathisia, insomnia, nausea, fatigue, restlessness and dry mouth. In controlled conditions, aripiprazole was not found to be effective for the treatment of acute depressive episodes in BD type I.[34]

Cariprazine

Cariprazine, a recently approved novel antipsychotic, is a partial agonist at the D2R/D3R, with higher affinity for the latter receptor. It has already been approved for schizophrenia and the treatment of manic and mixed episodes of BD type I, while studies are ongoing for negative-symptom schizophrenia, MDD, and BD maintenance. In a trial that was recently published, cariprazine's efficacy was shown in acute BD type I depression. In this multicenter study, cases were randomized to either cariprazine monotherapy dosed at 0.75, 1.5 or 3 mg/d, or placebo. The primary and secondary efficacy parameters were change from baseline MADRS and CGI-BP scores, respectively, and data were analyzed using a mixed effects model for repeated measures on the adjusted intent-to-treat population. At week 6, cariprazine 1.5 mg/d was statistically better than placebo on the primary, as well as secondary, efficacy measures, whereas the other two doses were not significantly different from placebo. The most common adverse events with cariprazine ($\geq$10%) were akathisia and insomnia, while weight gain was slightly higher with active treatment compared to placebo. In this rigorously conducted study, cariprazine mono-therapy showed consistent efficacy against bipolar depression and maintained a good tolerability and safety profile.[35]

Conclusion

BD is characterized by two extremes of illness: mania and depression. Whereas the manic pole of the ailment tends to be of shorter duration and typically responsive to the existing psychopharmacological agents, the depressive phase is often prolonged and poorly controlled by the currently available medications. The latter may express as MDEs, persisting sub-syn-dromal symptoms or mixed presentations in concurrence with manic mani-festations. The high risk of suicide is attributable to depressive symptoms and is further enhanced by the existence of mixed states and neuropsychiatric comorbidities such as anxiety and substance use disorders. Antidepressant monotherapy is often ineffective, and may worsen the prognosis by inducing mixed states, manic/hypomanic switches and rapid cycling. Further, classical mood stabilizers are not efficacious in a substantial number of cases. In this situation, there is an immediate need for better and more efficacious treat-ments. In the present chapter, the foremost psychotropic drugs for bipolar depression have been discussed to inform the modern management of this chronic ailment and evidence-based options are highlighted. It is hoped that with this knowledge, clinicians will be better able to deal with an otherwise intractable condition.

Summary Points

- BD is a chronic affective ailment in which there may be acute exacerba-tions or relatively quiescent periods with subthreshold symptoms.
- Whereas the manic episodes are circumscribed and typically remit with modern psychopharmacological agents, depressive episodes are more per-sistent and often resistent to treatment.
- The main burden of the disease is represented by depressive manifesta-tions which may be in the form of MDEs, mixed states or sub-syndromal symptoms.
- The disease burden is typified by psychosocial impairments at the one end, and recurrent acts of self-harm or completed suicides at the other extreme.
- Notably, general medical comorbidities add to the morbidity and mortality.
- Standard antidepressant medications are contraindicated as monotherapy in bipolar depression and are liable for mood destabilization.
- Monotherapy with conventional mood stabilizers like lithium and valpro-ate are often ineffective in treating patients with severe and complicated presentations.

- In this scenario there is an unmet need for new treatments that can alleviate the burden of bipolar depression and its associated comorbidities.
- Newer anticonvulsants and second and third generation antipsychotics are emerging as the mainstay of treatment of this intractable ailment.
- The recent approval of novel agents like cariprazine and brexpiprazole has provided new impetus for finding better cures for bipolar depression.

References

1) Ghaemi SN, Dalley S. The bipolar spectrum: conceptions and misconceptions. Aust N Z J Psychiatry 2014;48:314–324.
2) Dell'Aglio JC Jr, Basso LA, Argimon II, Arteche A. Systematic review of the prevalence of bipolar disorder and bipolar spectrum disorders in population-based studies. Trends Psychiatry Psychother 2013;35:99–105.
3) Hafeman DM, Merranko J, Axelson D, Goldstein BI, Goldstein T, Monk K, et al. Toward the definition of a bipolar prodrome: dimensional predictors of bipolar spectrum disorders in at-risk youths. Am J Psychiatry 2016;173:695–704.
4) Vieta E, Valentí M. Pharmacological management of bipolar depression: acute treatment, maintenance, and prophylaxis. CNS Drugs 2013;27:515–529.
5) Goldberg JF, Harrow M. A 15-year prospective follow-up of bipolar affective disorders: comparisons with unipolar nonpsychotic depression. Bipolar Disord 2011;13:155–163.
6) Citrome L. Treatment of bipolar depression: making sensible decisions. CNS Spectr 2014;19 Suppl 1:4–11.
7) Dell'Osso L, Del Grande C, Gesi C, Carmassi C, Musetti L. A new look at an old drug: neuroprotective effects and therapeutic potentials of lithium salts. Neuropsychiatr Dis Treat 2016;12:1687–1703.
8) Mulligan KA, Cheyette BN. Neurodevelopmental perspectives on Wnt signaling in psychiatry. Mol Neuropsychiatry 2017;2:219–246.
9) Stertz L, Fries GR, Aguiar BW, Pfaffenseller B, Valvassori SS, Gubert C, et al. Histone deacetylase activity and brain-derived neurotrophic factor (BDNF) levels in a pharmacological model of mania. Rev Bras Psiquiatr 2014;36:39–46.
10) Young AH, McElroy SL, Bauer M, Philips N, Chang W, Olausson B, et al. A double-blind, placebo-controlled study of quetiapine and lithium monotherapy in adults in the acute phase of bipolar depression (EMBOLDEN I). J Clin Psychiatry 2010;71:150–162.
11) Missio G, Moreno DH, Fernandes F, Bio DS, Soeiro-de-Souza MG, Rodrigues dos Santos D Jr, et al. The ARIQUELI study: potentiation of quetiapine in bipolar I nonresponders with lithium versus aripiprazole. Trials 2013;14:190.
12) Lewitzka U, Jabs B, Fülle M, Holthoff V, Juckel G, Uhl I, et al. Does lithium reduce acute suicidal ideation and behavior? A protocol for a randomized, placebo-controlled multicenter trial of lithium plus Treatment As Usual (TAU) in patients with suicidal major depressive episode. BMC Psychiatry 2015;15:117.
13) El-Mallakh RS, Salem MR, Chopra A, Mickus GJ, Penagaluri P, Movva R. A blinded, randomized comparison of immediate-release and extended-release carbamazepine capsules in manic and depressed bipolar subjects. Ann Clin Psychiatry 2010;22:3–8.

14) Juruena MF, Ottoni GL, Machado-Vieira R, Carneiro RM, Weingarthner N, Marquardt AR, et al. Bipolar I and II disorder residual symptoms: oxcarbazepine and carbamazepine as add-on treatment to lithium in a double-blind, randomized trial. Prog Neuropsychopharmacol Biol Psychiatry 2009;33:94–99.

15) Grunze H, Kotlik E, Costa R, Nunes T, Falcão A, Almeida L, et al. Assessment of the efficacy and safety of eslicarbazepine acetate in acute mania and prevention of recurrence: experience from multicentre, double-blind, randomised phase II clinical studies in patients with bipolar disorder I. J Affect Disord 2015;174:70–82.

16) Ghaemi SN, Gilmer WS, Goldberg JF, Zablotsky B, Kemp DE, Kelley ME, et al. Divalproex in the treatment of acute bipolar depression: a preliminary double-blind, randomized, placebo-controlled pilot study. J Clin Psychiatry 2007;68:1840–1844.

17) Muzina DJ, Gao K, Kemp DE, Khalife S, Ganocy SJ, Chan PK, et al. Acute efficacy of divalproex sodium versus placebo in mood stabilizer-naive bipolar I or II depression: a double-blind, randomized, placebo-controlled trial. J Clin Psychiatry 2011;72:813–819.

18) Bond DJ, Lam RW, Yatham LN. Divalproex sodium versus placebo in the treatment of acute bipolar depression: a systematic review and meta-analysis. J Affect Disord 2010;124:228–34.

19) Calabrese JR, Huffman RF, White RL, Edwards S, Thompson TR, Ascher JA, et al. Lamotrigine in the acute treatment of bipolar depression: results of five double-blind, placebo-controlled clinical trials. Bipolar Disord 2008;10:323–333.

20) Pigott K, Galizia I, Vasudev K, Watson S, Geddes J, Young AH. Topiramate for acute affective episodes in bipolar disorder in adults. Cochrane Database Syst Rev 2016;9:CD003384.

21) Schaffer LC, Schaffer CB, Miller AR, Manley JL, Piekut JA, Nordahl TE. An open trial of pregabalin as an acute and maintenance adjunctive treatment for outpatients with treatment resistant bipolar disorder. J Affect Disord 2013;147:407–410.

22) Coplan JD, Aaronson CJ, Panthangi V, Kim Y. Treating comorbid anxiety and depression: psychosocial and pharmacological approaches. World J Psychiatry 2015;5:366–378.

23) Saricicek A, Maloney K, Muralidharan A, Ruf B, Blumberg HP, Sanacora G, et al. Levetiracetam in the management of bipolar depression: a randomized, double-blind, placebo-controlled trial. J Clin Psychiatry 2011;72:744–750.

24) de Bartolomeis A, Tomasetti C, Iasevoli F. Update on the mechanism of action of aripiprazole: translational insights into antipsychotic strategies beyond dopamine receptor antagonism. CNS Drugs 2015;29:773–799.

25) Macfadden W, Adler CM, Turkoz I, Haskins JT, Turner N, Alphs L. Adjunctive long-acting risperidone in patients with bipolar disorder who relapse frequently and have active mood symptoms. BMC Psychiatry 2011;11:171.

26) Fu DJ, Turkoz I, Simonson RB, Walling DP, Schooler NR, Lindenmayer JP, et al. Paliperidone palmitate once-monthly reduces risk of relapse of psychotic, depressive, and manic symptoms and maintains functioning in a double-blind, randomized study of schizoaffective disorder. J Clin Psychiatry 2015;76:253–262.

27) Tohen M, Katagiri H, Fujikoshi S, Kanba S. Efficacy of olanzapine monotherapy in acute bipolar depression: a pooled analysis of controlled studies. J Affect Disord 2013;149:196–201.

28) Tohen M, Vieta E, Calabrese J, Ketter TA, Sachs G, Bowden C, et al. Efficacy of olanzapine and olanzapine-fluoxetine combination in the treatment of bipolar I depression. Arch Gen Psychiatry 2003;60:1079–1088.

29) Suttajit S, Srisurapanont M, Maneeton N, Maneeton B. Quetiapine for acute bipolar depression: a systematic review and meta-analysis. Drug Des Devel Ther 2014;8:827–838.

30) Lombardo I, Sachs G, Kolluri S, Kremer C, Yang R. Two 6-week, randomized, double-blind, placebo-controlled studies of ziprasidone in outpatients with bipolar I depression: did baseline characteristics impact trial outcome? J Clin Psychopharmacol 2012;32:470–478.

31) Sachs GS, Ice KS, Chappell PB, Schwartz JH, Gurtovaya O, Vanderburg DG, et al. Efficacy and safety of adjunctive oral ziprasidone for acute treatment of depression in patients with bipolar I disorder: a randomized, double-blind, placebo-controlled trial. J Clin Psychiatry 2011;72:1413–1422.

32) Loebel A, Cucchiaro J, Silva R, Kroger H, Hsu J, Sarma K, et al. Lurasidone monotherapy in the treatment of bipolar I depression: a randomized, double-blind, placebo-controlled study. Am J Psychiatry 2014;171:160–168.

33) Loebel A, Cucchiaro J, Silva R, Kroger H, Sarma K, Xu J, et al. Lurasidone as adjunctive therapy with lithium or valproate for the treatment of bipolar I depression: a randomized, double-blind, placebo-controlled study. Am J Psychiatry 2014;171:169–177.

34) Thase ME, Jonas A, Khan A, Bowden CL, Wu X, McQuade RD, et al. Aripiprazole monotherapy in nonpsychotic bipolar I depression: results of 2 randomized, placebo-controlled studies. J Clin Psychopharmacol 2008;28:13–20.

35) Durgam S, Earley W, Lipschitz A, Guo H, Laszlovszky I, Németh G, et al. An 8-week randomized, double-blind, placebo-controlled evaluation of the safety and efficacy of cariprazine in patients with bipolar I depression. Am J Psychiatry 2016;173:271–281.

36) Gabriel A. Adjunctive topiramate treatment in refractory obese bipolar patients: a descriptive open label study. Eat Weight Disord 2007;12:48–53.

37) Wang PW, Santosa C, Scumacher M, Winsberg ME, Strong C, Ketter TA. Gabapentin augmentation therapy in bipolar depression. Bipolar Disord 2002;4:296–301.

10 Manic Phase of Bipolar Disorder

Treatment Recommendations

Introduction

The presence of mania defines bipolarity and as such its accurate diagnosis and treatment is central to the successful long-term management of bipolar disorder (BD). Clinically, BD usually presents with depressive symptoms that are indistinguishable from those of major depressive disorder (MDD), and because of this overlap it is often misdiagnosed at the outset, and only when manic/hypomanic symptoms emerge, does the illness declare itself. In practice, this delays diagnosis, often considerably (4–10 years), and in the interim patients may receive suboptimal treatment that worsens their prognosis[1]. As BD has been re-conceptualized as a lifelong disease instead of an episodic illness, there has been greater emphasis on long-term management. This change has shifted the focus of management from the treatment of acute episodes towards that of prevention and the maintenance of well-being, and in this regard the development of specific psychological interventions in conjunction with prophylactic pharmacotherapies have played an important role. However, psychological treatments are most beneficial when administered during periods of remission, and thus in reality, only individuals that are relatively well in the first place are able to obtain access and gain benefit from them.[2]

This chapter briefly discusses the diagnosis of mania, upon which the characterization of BD type I (BD I) is based, and considers the recommendations for its management by incorporating the evidence from the most up-to-date treatment guidelines.

Diagnosis of Mania

Mania is the *sine qua non* of the bipolar diathesis, and Figure 10.1 summarizes the signs and symptoms of this disturbance in an illustrated manner.

Mania is a distinct period of abnormally and persistently elevated, expansive or irritable mood, lasting at least one week and is accompanied by marked psychosocial impairment.To meet the Diagnostic and Statistical Manual of Mental Disorders – 5th Edition (DSM-5) criteria for a manic episode patients must additionally have at least four of the following symptoms:[3]

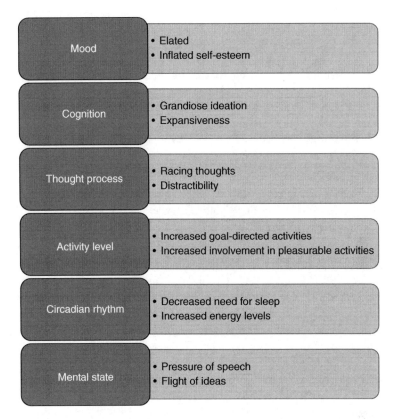

Figure 10.1 Features of mania according to different symptom domains

The occurrence of at least one manic episode is required for the diagnosis of bipolar disorder (BD) type I. This schematic illustrates the cardinal manifestations of mania, upon which the diagnosis of the diathesis is made. The duration of the disturbance should be one week, but this stipulation is set aside if the patient needs hospitalization.

a) inflated self-esteem or grandiosity,
b) decreased need for sleep,
c) pressured speech,
d) racing thoughts,
e) distractibility,
f) increased goal-directed activity or psychomotor agitation, and
g) excessive involvement in pleasurable activities with a high potential for adverse consequences.

In practice, the diagnosis of florid sustained mania is relatively straightforward but the diagnosis of less severe forms such as hypomania can be difficult as patients usually manifest observable clinical symptoms but without significant functional impairment. Further, many individuals often experience elevated mood as ego syntonic, and therefore do not consider their hypomanic symptoms as problematic and often fail to seek help. In addition, when hypomanic symptoms occur interspersed within protracted periods of depression that are common in BD type II, patients understandably find it difficult to recognize euthymia and therefore regard their hypomanic episodes as normal, mainly because these symptoms are often enjoyable and seemingly productive and therefore preferable to depression.[4] Regardless, the treatment of both mania and hypomania is essentially with similar agents, albeit the dosage of the medications employed may vary according to the severity of the presentation.

Treatment of Mania

Current Treatment Guidelines for Bipolar Disorder

Since 2009 several national and international BD treatment guidelines have been published which include the International College of Neuro-Psychopharmacology (CINP), the Canadian Network for Mood and Anxiety Treatments (CANMAT), the World Federation of Societies of Biological Psychiatry (WFSBP), the British Association for Psychopharmacology (BAP) and the National Institute for Health and Care Excellence (NICE). Treatment guidelines serve a useful purpose as they summarize the evidence available for management pathways. However, recommendations can vary substantially, as every guideline develops its own methodology and unique criteria for evaluating the extant literature. Consequently, although the various treatment guidelines in essence examine the "same evidence", because they adopt diverse approaches the resulting recommendations have notable differences.[5] Though the consensus ratings evaluate a wide range of findings summarized within the guidelines, there is considerable additional evidence in the form of case reports and open studies that is usually not incorporated. As such, because of this limitation there are unavoidable gaps that cannot be addressed. Guidelines additionally do not capture the vast array of variables that impact clinical choice including past history, family history of response, tolerability issues, comorbidity and personal preference. Therefore it is important to appreciate that these recommendations can only provide a general direction and for meaningful application, have to be used in the broader context of clinical experience.[6] Figure 10.2 is a diagrammatic rendition of the pharmacotherapy of acute mania as endorsed by the latest versions of highly acclaimed practice guidelines.

Pharmacotherapy of Acute Mania

Acute mania often results in loss of insight, behavioral disturbance and risky behavior. In these instances, the least restrictive care environment compatible with secure management is chosen, and medication is often the only option for safe and immediate treatment.[7] A broad range of "antimanic"

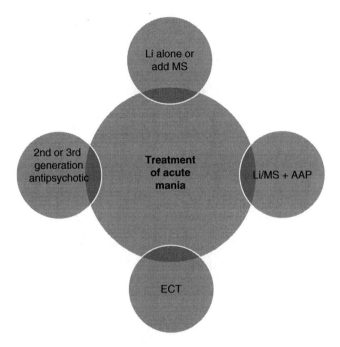

Figure 10.2 Pharmacotherapy of acute mania in bipolar disorder type I

The latest versions of widely acclaimed treatment guidelines for bipolar disorder (BD) recommend that acute mania be controlled with an atypical antipsychotic (AAP), preferably as monotherapy. There is good evidence of efficacy for several second (quetiapine, olanzapine) and third (aripiprazole, cariprazine) generation antipsychotics. The use of lithium (Li) or anticonvulsant mood stabilizers (MS) either alone or in combination is no longer considered first-line. In difficult to manage cases Li or MS can be combined with AAP. Lastly, electroconvulsive therapy (ECT) is reserved for treatment refractory mania.

medications for mania/hypomania are currently available. These include second and third generation antipsychotics, anticonvulsants and lithium.[8] As first-line, monotherapy is the ideal, and for nonpsychotic manic episodes there is unanimous consensus across the guidelines with respect to mood stabilizers (MS), i.e., lithium and valproate. The atypical antipsychotics olanzapine, risperidone, quetiapine, ziprasidone and aripiprazole also achieve a consensus recommendation of first-line therapy, even though olanzapine and quetiapine are both regarded as second-line by the WFSBP guidelines, because of their long-term unfavorable side effect profiles.[9] In the short-term management of acute mania tolerability is perhaps less critical, with the caveat that successful acute therapy often becomes long-term by default. Further, atypical antipsychotics (AAP) do offer some advantages, such as intramuscular administration, which is sometimes necessary when there is pronounced behavioral agitation. Interestingly, lithium is ranked highly, and clearly it has a robust evidence base for its efficacy.

However, because of its relatively slow onset of action it is seldom used as monotherapy in the acute setting and an adjunctive antipsychotic agent is often used for rapid symptomatic relief and control of behavioral disturbance.[10] The armamentarium has increased in this regard with recently published RCTs endorsing the role of asenapine, paliperidone and cariprazine in acute manic and mixed episodes.[11] Combination therapy (MS + AAP) is often necessary when symptoms are not adequately controlled with a single first-line agent and this is more likely in severe or psychotic mania, or that accompanied by behavioral disturbance. The following steps are recommended in the control of acute mania:[12]

First step:

- Discontinue treatment with antidepressants.
- Start with aripiprazole, asenapine, cariprazine, paliperidone, quetiapine or risperidone monotherapy.
- If the patient is already under one of the above first-step monotherapy and response is unsatisfactory, switch to another first-step monotherapy.

Second step:

If the interventions recommended during the first step fail or the response is unsatisfactory, then apply:

- Olanzapine or ziprasidone monotherapy.
- Combinations of lithium or valproate plus an AAP.
- Lithium or valproate plus a first generation antipsychotic (FGA), e.g., haloperidol.

Third step:

- Apply electroconvulsive therapy (ECT) on top of pharmacological treatment.
- Switch to oxcarbazepine as a MS.

Fourth step:

- Various combinations of medication according to anecdotal knowledge or the personal experience of the therapist.

Many of the agents considered as second-line (carbamazepine, haloperidol, pimozide) demonstrate reasonable efficacy but are considered to be secondary because of poor tolerability. Amongst these, the BAP guidelines recommend carbamazepine first-line but acknowledge its potential for drug interaction and therefore overall, it has been relegated to second-line administration. Similarly, the evidence for the combination of lithium and valproate is promising but stems predominantly from uncontrolled trials and therefore both CANMAT and WFSBP guidelines have assigned it second-line status and the CINP recommends its use for refractory mania.[13]

Therapies ranked as third-line or lower still, usually lack evidence, have been shown to be less efficacious or have a poor side effect profile. As a consequence, clinical experience with these agents is also often lacking. For example, clozapine has received varying recommendations. As monotherapy it is not as efficacious as other medications and has an adverse side effect profile. Hence the WFSBP guidelines recommend its use fourth-line; however, because of evidence for its adjunctive use in refractory illness it is reasonable to consider its administration earlier, as a third-line option.[14]

The combination of lithium and haloperidol is recommended third-line by the CINP and CANMAT guidelines mainly because of poor tolerability. However, the regimen has proven efficacy in mania and for this reason BAP and NICE have positioned it first- and second-line respectively. Largely, given the many other options with AAP a third-line recommendation is considered unsuitable. The combination of lithium and carbamazepine has both lower efficacy than first-line therapies and greater adverse side effects, and therefore the CINP guidelines recommend this combination as second-line, ideally for refractory illness, and CANMAT suggests third-line usage. Hence overall, both of these combinations have been placed as third-line because of their poor tolerability, which is an important consideration especially if treatment is to be continued in the long term as is often the case in clinical practice.[15] Interestingly, ECT is also recommended third-line with consensus across the guidelines, and the WFSBP guidelines specify its use for "severe delirious mania" or refractory mania when adequate trials of first- and second-line therapies have been exhausted.[16]

Pharmacological agents that clearly lack antimanic efficacy (e.g., lamotrigine) are not indicated in mania, and combinations that cause significant side effects, such as carbamazepine with haloperidol, are not advisable. Following on from the success of agents such as valproate and carbamazepine, a number of anticonvulsants (topiramate, gabapentin, levetiracetam and eslicarbazepine) have been tested in controlled trials unsuccessfully and are therefore not recommended by any of the guidelines. Similarly, other agents investigated for the treatment of mania such as pregabalin, zonisamide and tiagabine have accrued insufficient evidence and are therefore either considered as fourth-line therapies or not recommended at all.

Finally, brief mention of a recent meta-analysis is necessary because of its rigor and likely impact on future treatment guidelines and clinical practice. Specifically, it found haloperidol and the AAP risperidone, olanzapine and quetiapine were significantly more effective than lithium, valproate and carbamazepine.[17] Effectiveness included both efficacy (change in YMRS at week 3) and acceptability (drop out by week 3) but only evaluated short-term outcome (day 21) and, therefore, the findings have been criticized for not emphasizing enough how these rankings would change if treatment was continued long-term. Other meta-analyses using different rankings have come up with quite divergent findings.[18]

Management Issues

The pharmacological agents chosen to treat acute mania should be determined by the clinical presentation of the episode. For instance, in classic euphoric mania lithium is indicated, while valproate is more appropriate in mixed mania. With severe presentations and accompanying psychotic symptoms, an AAP should be chosen. In all cases, any ongoing antidepressant medication should be ceased immediately. Further, adherence to continuing treatment should be confirmed and when possible, serum levels should be monitored to ensure therapeutic levels. For example, levels lower than 0.6 mmol/L for lithium are likely to result in poorer acute response and a greater risk of relapse. Additionally, side effects should be carefully monitored while increasing the dosage or adding medication. Patients who have not been on treatment previously require special consideration. Ideally, a first-line treatment should be initiated and optimized while monitoring efficacy and tolerability/adherence. Generally, medications take one to two weeks at therapeutic plasma levels to take effect, and if symptoms persist after two weeks at adequate levels, the patient is unlikely to respond. In such instances, other first-line treatments or combinations may be tried, followed by second- and third-line treatments if necessary. Further, patients who have significant behavioral disturbance may require treatment with a parenteral antipsychotic medication. In patients with severe symptoms who are failing to respond, ECT merits consideration.[19]

Maintenance Treatment

General Considerations

Theoretically, maintenance treatment begins after a significant period of mood stability has been achieved following an acute episode. However, there is no clear consensus on what constitutes acute treatment and how this evolves to maintenance therapy with resulting difficulties when attempting to compare research studies. In addition to this, many of the endpoints used to evaluate effectiveness of maintenance treatment (such as number, length and severity of episodes) have been measured variably by different research groups. Therefore, much of the research into this critical treatment phase of the disorder is challenging to evaluate and integrate meaningfully.[20] BD by its very nature is a chronic illness with frequent relapses; therefore, it is increasingly apparent that achieving symptom remission is simply inadequate. For example, a well-cited naturalistic effectiveness study found that 40% of patients who had recovered from a manic or mixed episode necessitating hospitalization, experienced a relapse within two years.[21] Hence, maintenance therapy is critical as it protects against relapse by reducing the number, intensity and length of episodes, and by treating inter-episode symptoms. Importantly, it also diminishes suicide rates and improves psychosocial functioning. However, a key difficulty with maintenance therapy is that of acceptance of the presence of illness, the need for ongoing treatment and adherence to medications.[22]

Psychological Therapy

Psychological interventions are a crucial component of maintenance therapy and have benefits above and beyond medications that lead to better and more sustained recovery. They are therefore recommended for the management of BD alongside pharmacotherapy wherever possible. Specifically, psychological interventions have been shown to effectively reduce the likelihood of relapse, mood fluctuations and decrease the need for medications and hospitalization, while at the same time improving adherence to medication and global functioning.[23]

Interestingly, long-term psychological interventions tend to be more effective for depression than mania, and are more useful when used early in the course of the disorder. The components of most psychological therapies that contribute to their long-term success in maintaining mood include psychoeducation, the promotion of medication adherence, dealing with negative cognitions, mood monitoring and the regulation of daily activities and sleep.[24] Together, these facilitate the detection of early warning signs indicative of relapse and the use of coping strategies to deal with the potential recurrence of symptoms. The most widely used approaches in BD are psychoeducation (PE), cognitive behavioral therapy (CBT), interpersonal therapy (IPT) and family-focused therapy (FFT).

As the name suggests PE involves informing patients and/or families about BD and its course. Specifically, it emphasizes the importance of treatment adherence, the early detection of manic symptoms and the adoption of a structured lifestyle. PE can be delivered to patients individually or in a group setting, and can also involve caregivers. It is effective in reducing the length of acute episodes, hospitalizations and relapse rates. Recently, web-based PE programs have also shown promise in maintenance and are accessible and cost-effective. Hence, PE in maintenance is recommended first-line alongside pharmacotherapy.[25]

CBT provides structured therapy and teaches patients to identify links between cognitions, feelings and behaviors, and to understand how these result in clinical symptoms. Patients are taught to monitor thoughts, challenge dysfunctional beliefs and acquire coping skills. With maintenance CBT, most studies have shown a decrease in relapse and recurrence of mania, but to a lesser extent than for depression. Like PE, CBT is effective both individually and in group settings, and is highly recommended for maintenance therapy.[26]

IPT is also effective in lowering relapse and hospitalizations for both mania and depression, especially in those patients who have recently experienced an acute episode. In IPT, patients are taught to recognize how a change to their interpersonal environment (e.g., change in role, grief and loss) affects mood and then implement strategies to deal with these by building social skills to assist in problem solving. Current treatment guidelines recommend IPT as an adjunct to pharmacotherapy, particularly in the acute phase of the disorder and for the long-term prevention of depression.[27]

Finally, FFT provides families of patients with supportive therapy and equips them with skills to effectively manage the disorder. It too has been found to be efficacious in preventing relapse and recurrence, and again more so with depression than mania. Like other psychological interventions it is useful as an adjunctive therapy to pharmacological treatment. Selecting the type of psychological therapy to be used requires an inclusive approach, though interestingly the relapse rates in patients receiving PE or CBT appear to be similar. This is an important consideration given the cost of PE is about a third of the cost of the other, more structured psychotherapies which are best delivered by trained psychologists. PE, on the other hand, is clear-cut and the treating physician can offer it in an adequate manner alongside pharmacotherapy. Similarly, group-based programs have cost advantages over individual approaches; however there are no head-to-head studies comparing these options.

Pharmacotherapy

With long-term pharmacotherapy, safety and tolerability considerations are as important as efficacy. Hence, monotherapy is usually preferable as first-line treatment, and combination as second-line. Such recommendations are endorsed by CANMAT and BAP, whereas others (CINP and WFSBP) do not explicitly mention recommendations of specific combinations. The NICE guidelines acknowledge concerns of safety and tolerability but also point out that some combinations are possibly more efficacious than monotherapy.[28] Following an acute episode of illness (mania/depression) recurrence is highly probable and it is likely that maintenance treatment will be necessary life-long. The likelihood of relapse is high if there is a history of frequent relapses, psychotic episodes, comorbid substance abuse, stressful life events or poor social supports.

The efficacy of lithium in treating BD has been robustly demonstrated over the last 60 years and therefore it is commonly used as a comparator for newer medications. It is recommended first-line across all guidelines and its real-world effectiveness has been further demonstrated by the BALANCE Study, a large multi-site, international study.[29] Lithium is also unique as it is effective in reducing rates of suicide and may be neuroprotective. Valproate is also recommended as a first-line option by NICE and BAP, but because it is less efficacious than lithium the WFSBP and CINP have placed it as second-line. In comparison, lamotrigine is interesting because it is also recommended first-line for maintenance but it should be noted that it has specific effectiveness in BD type II and the prevention of depressive episodes rather than mania.[30] Hence, it would not be appropriate to prescribe lamotrigine if the patient has a predominantly manic pole of illness. With regards to antipsychotics, olanzapine and aripiprazole are recommended first-line and are particularly efficacious for mania. Quetiapine is also indicated first-line overall but is recommended in the CINP guideline as a second-line adjunctive treatment because it has good evidence in the depressive pole, and is particularly efficacious for the treatment of BD type II.[31]

Carbamazepine and oxcarbazepine are not as efficacious as lithium in maintenance treatment and due to their adverse side effects most guidelines place them second-line. Further, the CANMAT guidelines recommend oxcarbazepine adjunctively as third-line therapy. Risperidone has demonstrated efficacy in preventing manic relapse and can also be administered as a long-acting injection. It is recommended as first-line by CANMAT both as monotherapy and as an adjunct. Nevertheless, the CINP and WFSBP guidelines place it as third- and fourth-line respectively. However, in light of recent research it has been placed as second-line overall.[32] With regards to ziprasidone the CINP has placed it third-line as the evidence was evaluated as lacking, but the CANMAT guidelines favor its use as an adjunctive therapy. Hence overall it has been placed second-line.

As previously mentioned, most guidelines suggest combination therapy in maintenance as second-line. The most commonly mentioned combinations are lithium or valproate and an antipsychotic such as risperidone, olanzapine, quetiapine or aripiprazole. Other combinations that have been recommended include lithium or valproate plus lamotrigine, lithium plus valproate, olanzapine plus fluoxetine, and lithium or valproate plus carbamazepine. Of note however, BAP does not recommend carbamazepine be combined with other therapies due to drug interactions. According to the evidence evaluated by each of the guidelines, these combinations confer reasonable prophylaxis, and the NICE guidelines have placed combination therapies as first-line. However, one of the most important considerations of multiple medications regimen long-term is that of tolerability and adverse side effects, which would potentially reduce adherence.[33] Clozapine is recommended unanimously by most guidelines as third-line monotherapy, or adjunctive therapy. Interestingly, it remains widely used in maintenance even though there is an absence of randomized controlled trials and clinically it requires regular monitoring for side effects.

A final note about the recent developments in the maintenance treatment of chronic psychiatric ailments including BD, schizoaffective disorders and schizophrenia. Pilot open-label studies and controlled trials have demonstrated the efficacy and safety of long-acting injectable formulations of AAP. The use of these agents is widely advocated, and in actual practice there are significant advantages. For instance, adherence is ensured, patients experience fewer relapses and exhibit better psychosocial functioning. The medications already available include long-acting preparations of risperidone, paliperidone, olanzapine and aripiprazole which are administered intramuscularly

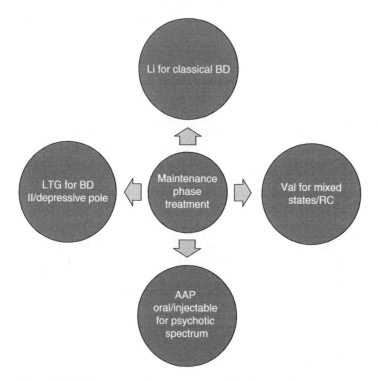

Figure 10.3 Maintenance phase treatment of bipolar disorder

Bipolar disorder (BD) is a chronic condition with high rates of recurrence, and therefore main-tenance treatment is a priority. BD patients can exhibit the whole spectrum of affective symp-tomatology with recurrent manic, depressive or mixed episodes and rapid cycling. Additionally, psychotic symptoms commonly occur during the course of any severe episode. In this scenario while lithium (Li) is efficacious as maintenance therapy in classical BD, valproate (Val) is more effective in mixed episodes and rapid cycling (RC). Lamotrigine's (LTG) effectiveness as a main-tenance agent is limited to BD type II and patients with predominantly depressive recurrences. Atypical antipsychotics (AAP), oral and injectable, are emerging as first-line medications in BD with psychotic features and schizoaffective disorders.

once every two to four weeks. With accumulating clinical experience, it is very likely such medications would assume first-line status in the maintenance treatment of psychiatric patients with chronic disorders.[34] Figure 10.3 gives a schematic representation of the foremost medications used in the mainte-nance treatment of BD, and emphasizes the importance of lithium, anticon-vulsant mood stabilizers and atypical antipsychotics.

Conclusion

BD is a lifelong illness and carries a high rate of mortality which arises from an increased risk of suicide and general medical comorbidities. Quintessentially, it is defined by the occurrence of mania and a range of pharmacological agents are presently available to treat both acute exacerbations and maintain long-term prophylaxis. For acute mania, pharmacotherapy is the pivotal treatment, with the aim of rapid symptom relief as well as the management of behavioral/psychotic disturbance. In this respect, current guidelines recommend second and third generation antipsychotics either alone or in conjunction with first-line mood stabilizers. However, given the chronic recurrent nature of the illness, it is imperative clinicians keep maintenance treatment in mind when considering options for acute pharmacotherapy. The primary goal of long-term management is maintenance of euthymic mood and prevention of future episodes. Effective long-term treatment requires a combination of pharmacological, lifestyle and psychological interventions. In the clinical setting denial of the illness, inadequate knowledge of the disorder and its treatment, and the long-term tolerability of the medications employed, are issues that often lead to poor adherence and relapse. In this regard psychological interventions, particularly psychoeducation have been found to be valuable. Interestingly, despite the expanding evidence for the effectiveness of psychological and pharmacological therapies, the majority of patients continue to experience recurrence despite receiving recommended treatment. With the present gaps in the knowledge regarding the pathophysiology of this disorder and the absence of curative treatments, the optimal strategy is adherence to the biopsychosocial model, which should be followed to alleviate the challenges imposed by the bipolar diathesis.

Summary Points

- Mania and depression are the two opposing mood states of the bipolar diathesis.
- Manic episodes are a psychiatric emergency, requiring immediate control in a safe and secure environment.
- Substantial progress has been made in the acute pharmacotherapy of manic exacerbations.
- In this regard, the management should be according to the recommendations of comprehensive evidence-based guidelines issued by eminent organizations.
- In the present chapter a brief outline is provided with the focus on acute mania and prophylactic treatment.
- In the light of controlled trials, a clearer picture is emerging and has the endorsement of influential international guidelines.
- The foremost conclusion is that second and third generation antipsychotics are most important not only in the control of acute mania, but also their long-acting injectable formulations are poised to play the same role in the maintenance treatment of BD.
- Since patients continue to have relapses in spite of best possible treatment, there is an urgent need for novel medications that are curative rather than palliative in nature.

References

1) Fritz K, Russell AMT, Allwang C, Kuiper S, Lampe L, Malhi GS. Is a delay in the diagnosis of bipolar disorder inevitable? Bipolar Disord 2017;[Epub ahead of print].

2) Scott J, Etain B. Which psychosocial interventions in bipolar depression? Encephale 2011;37 Suppl 3:S214–217.

3) Kaltenboeck A, Winkler D, Kasper S. Bipolar and related disorders in DSM-5 and ICD-10. CNS Spectr 2016;21:318–323.

4) Dubovsky SL. Mania. Continuum (MinneapMinn) 2015;21:737–755.

5) Parker GB, Graham RK, Tavella G. Is there consensus across international evidence-based guidelines for the management of bipolar disorder? ActaPsychiatrScand 2017;135:515–526.

6) Samalin L, Llorca PM. Methodological approach to inter "guideline" variability in the management of bipolar disorders. Encephale 2012;38:126–132.[Article in French]

7) Grande I, Vieta E. Pharmacotherapy of acute mania: monotherapy or combination therapy with mood stabilizers and antipsychotics? CNS Drugs 2015;29:221–227.

8) Ogawa Y, Tajika A, Takeshima N, Hayasaka Y, Furukawa TA. Mood stabilizers and antipsychotics for acute mania: a systematic review and meta-analysis of combination/augmentation therapy versus monotherapy. CNS Drugs 2014;28:989–1003.

9) Grunze H, Vieta E, Goodwin GM, Bowden C, Licht RW, Moller HJ, et al. The World Federation of Societies of Biological Psychiatry (WFSBP) guidelines for the biological treatment of bipolar disorders: update 2009 on the treatment of acute mania. World J Biol Psychiatry 2009;10:85–116.

10) Samalin L, Guillaume S, Courtet P, Abbar M, Lancrenon S, Llorca PM. Methodological differences between pharmacological treatment guidelines for bipolar disorder: what to do for the clinicians? Compr Psychiatry 2013;54:309–320.

11) Calabrese JR, Keck PE Jr, Starace A, Lu K, Ruth A, Laszlovszky I, et al. Efficacy and safety of low- and high-dose cariprazine in acute and mixed mania associated with bipolar I disorder: a double-blind, placebo-controlled study. J Clin Psychiatry 2015;76:284–292.

12) Fountoulakis KN, Grunze H, Vieta E, Young A, Yatham L, Blier P, et al. The International College of Neuro-Psychopharmacology (CINP) treatment guidelines for bipolar disorder in adults (CINP-BD-2017), part 3: the clinical guidelines. Int J Neuropsychopharmacol 2017; 20: 180–195.

13) Yatham LN, Kennedy SH, Parikh SV, Schaffer A, Beaulieu S, Alda M, et al. Canadian Network for Mood and Anxiety Treatments (CANMAT) and International Society for Bipolar Disorders (ISBD) collaborative update of CANMAT guidelines for the management of patients with bipolar disorder: update 2013. Bipolar Disord 2013;15:1–44.

14) Grunze H, Vieta E, Goodwin GM, Bowden C, Licht RW, Möller HJ, et al. The World Federation of Societies of Biological Psychiatry (WFSBP) guidelines for the biological treatment of bipolar disorders: update 2012 on the long-term treatment of bipolar disorder.World J Biol Psychiatry 2013;14:154–219.

15) Morriss R. Mandatory implementation of NICE Guidelines for the care of bipolar disorder and other conditions in England and Wales. BMC Med 2015;13:246.

16) Jacobowski NL, Heckers S, Bobo WV. Delirious mania: detection, diagnosis, and clinical management in the acute setting. J PsychiatrPract 2013;19:15–28.

17) Yildiz A, Nikodem M, Vieta E, Correll CU, Baldessarini RJ. A network meta-analysis on comparative efficacy and all-cause discontinuation of antimanic treatments in acute bipolar mania. Psychol Med 2015;45:299–317.

18) Goikolea JM, Colom F, Capapey J, Torres I, Valenti M, Grande I, et al. Faster onset of antimanic action with haloperidol compared to second-generation antipsychotics. A meta-analysis of randomized clinical trials in acute mania. Eur Neuropsychopharmacol 2013;23:305–316.

19) Nivoli AM, Murru A, Goikolea JM, Crespo JM, Montes JM, González-Pinto A, et al. New treatment guidelines for acute bipolar mania: a critical review. J Affect Disord 2012;140:125–141.

20) Lindström L, Lindström E, Nilsson M, Höistad M. Maintenance therapy with second generation antipsychotics for bipolar disorder – a systematic review and meta-analysis. J Affect Disord 2017;213:138–150.

21) Tohen M, Zarate CA Jr, Hennen J, Khalsa HM, Strakowski SM, Gebre-Medhin P, et al. The McLean-Harvard First-Episode Mania Study: prediction of recovery and first recurrence. Am J Psychiatry 2003;160:2099–2107.

22) Samalin L, Nourry A, Charpeaud T, Llorca PM. What is the evidence for the use of second-generation antipsychotic long-acting injectables as maintenance treatment in bipolar disorder? Nord J Psychiatry 2014;68:227–235.

23) Husain MI, Chaudhry IB, Rahman RR, Hamirani MM, Mehmood N, Haddad PM, et al. Pilot study of a culturally adapted psychoeducation (CaPE) intervention for bipolar disorder in Pakistan. Int J Bipolar Disord 2017;5:3.

24) Haynes PL, Gengler D, Kelly M. Social rhythm therapies for mood disorders: an update. Curr Psychiatry Rep 2016;18:75.

25) Bond K, Anderson IM. Psychoeducation for relapse prevention in bipolar disorder: a systematic review of efficacy in randomized controlled trials. Bipolar Disord 2015;17:349–362.

26) Chiang KJ, Tsai JC, Liu D, Lin CH, Chiu HL, Chou KR. Efficacy of cognitive-behavioral therapy in patients with bipolar disorder: a meta-analysis of randomized controlled trials. PLoS One 2017;12:e0176849.

27) Swartz HA, Rucci P, Thase ME, Wallace M, Carretta E, Celedonia KL, et al. Psychotherapy alone and combined with medication as treatments for bipolar II depression: a randomized controlled trial. J Clin Psychiatry 2017;[Epub ahead of print].

28) Ostacher MJ, Tandon R, Suppes T. Florida best practice psychotherapeutic medication guidelines for adults with bipolar disorder: a novel, practical, patient-centered guide for clinicians. J Clin Psychiatry 2016;77:920–926.

29) BALANCE investigators and collaborators, Geddes JR, Goodwin GM, Rendell J, Azorin JM, Cipriani A, et al. Lithium plus valproate combination therapy versus monotherapy for relapse prevention in bipolar I disorder (BALANCE): a randomised open-label trial. Lancet 2010;375:385–395.

30) Gitlin M, Frye MA. Maintenance therapies in bipolar disorders. Bipolar Disord 2012;14:51–65.

31) Atkin T, Nuñez N, Gobbi G. Practitioner Review: the effects of atypical antipsychotics and mood stabilisers in the treatment of depressive symptoms in paediatric bipolar disorder. J Child Psychol Psychiatry 2017;58:865–879.

32) Yatham LN, Beaulieu S, Schaffer A, Kauer-Sant'Anna M, Kapczinski F, Lafer B, et al. Optimal duration of risperidone or olanzapine adjunctive therapy to mood stabilizer following remission of a manic episode: a CANMAT randomized double-blind trial. Mol Psychiatry 2016;21:1050–1056.

33) Fountoulakis KN, Yatham L, Grunze H, Vieta E, Young A, Blier P, et al. The International College of Neuro-Psychopharmacology (CINP) treatment guidelines for bipolar disorder in adults (CINP-BD-2017), part 2: review, grading of the evidence, and a precise algorithm. Int J Neuropsychopharmacol 2017;20:121–179.

34) Fountoulakis KN, Vieta E, Young A, Yatham L, Grunze H, Blier P, et al. The International College of Neuropsychopharmacology (CINP) treatment guidelines for bipolar disorder in adults (CINP-BD-2017), part 4: unmet needs in the treatment of bipolar disorder and recommendations for future research. Int J Neuropsychopharmacol 2017;20:196–205.

11 Non-Pharmacological Treatments for Mood Disorders

Psychological Treatments

Introduction

Mood disorders are exemplified by affective episodes which could be either depressive or manic in nature. Major depressive disorder (MDD) and the less severe but more chronic dysthymic disorder involve depressive exacerbations only, whereas bipolar disorder (BD) requires episodes of mania or hypomania. Mood disorders are among the most prevalent of psychiatric disorders, account for the vast majority of suicides and are a leading cause of disability in the psychosocial spheres of functioning.[1] The acute and long-term treatment of mood disorders is primarily with medications, however, three evidence-based non-pharmacological modalities are considered here and include manualized psychotherapies, electroconvulsive therapy and chronobiological techniques. These are schematically given in Figure 11.1.

Both psychotherapy and medications are widely used in the treatment of mood disorders. Historically, the primary focus of treatment development was on symptom reduction, but there has been a growing recognition of the need to develop strategies that prevent subsequent relapse and recurrence. Medication treatment has long been considered the standard of treatment for more severe depression and BD and has gained market share relative to psychotherapy in recent years with the advent of less problematic medications.

Nonetheless, non-adherence to pharmacotherapy is common, increasing the probability of recurrence and associated negative consequences. Patients often experience disruptive side effects, especially metabolic disturbance when taking second generation antipsychotics. Thus, adjunctive psychosocial interventions are increasingly used for mood disorders. Addition of psychosocial interventions have been shown to improve outcomes because they teach patients strategies to manage mood instability. Evidence supporting the utility of psychotherapy to reduce the risk of relapse (as opposed to relieving acute affective episodes) in people with both BD and MDD has been particularly robust.[2]

This section describes the most recent studies of empirically based, manualized psychosocial interventions for mood disorders. In particular, the following

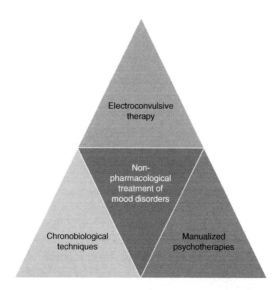

Figure 11.1 Non-pharmacological strategies for the treatment of mood disorders

Mood disorders are chronic, recalcitrant conditions with less than optimal response to pharmacotherapy in many cases. Additionally, many patients complain of adverse effects and have relative contraindications to psychotherapeutic medications. As such, non-pharmacological approaches are gaining in acceptance both by patients and clinicians. Three main practices are illustrated here, but see text for further details.

treatment modalities are examined: psychoeducation (PE), cognitive behavioral therapy (CBT), interpersonal and social rhythm therapy (IPSRT), dialectical behavior therapy (DBT), mindfulness-based cognitive behavioral therapy (MBCT), and family therapies such as family-focused therapy (FFT). Also discussed briefly are future areas of research to elucidate the current understanding of evidence-based treatments for major mood disorders. Accumulating evidence suggests psychotherapy can be an effective treatment for mood disorders when combined with pharmacotherapy.[3] Some psychotherapy techniques (e.g., PE, FFT, CBT) have been the focus of more randomized controlled studies whereas others have not (e.g., IPSRT, DBT, MBCT). The most promising strategies to date include PE, CBT and family therapies, with preliminary but positive findings for DBT and MBCT. These implications are schematically depicted in Figure 11.2 which summarizes the abovementioned arguments.

Psychoeducation

PE is a psychosocial approach that views mood disorders as medical conditions that would most significantly be improved with education about the diathesis, enabling patients to play a greater role in their treatment. PE is aimed at improving medication adherence and also includes strategies to enhance

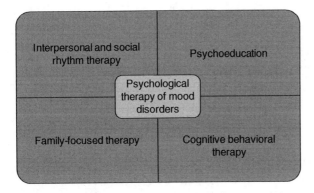

Figure 11.2 Evidence-based psychological therapy of mood disorders

Manualized psychotherapies which are limited in duration and number of sessions are an essential part of the overall management of patients with affective illnesses. The foremost techniques are depicted here, however, mindfulness-based cognitive therapy and dialectical behavior therapy are also gaining in acceptance.

awareness of triggers and associated problem solving strategies. PE encourages patients to be active participants in their own treatment and is often delivered in a group format.

PE has been associated with a longer time to mood episode recurrence and improved outpatient adherence to medication regimens, but may not be as effective as maintenance pharmacotherapy. PE does tend to be a more cost-effective intervention, since group (as opposed to individual) PE may be particularly efficacious. PE may also be more effective when administered in greater dose, i.e., more sessions of longer duration. In the past few years, online and mobile-based programs have been studied as an alternative means of delivering PE, with modest to poor efficacy.[4] However, online PE programs may be more effective when combined with online peer support or face-to-face sessions with a therapist.

Cognitive Behavioral Therapy

The focus of CBT is to modify dysfunctional thought patterns and behaviors. Furthermore, it aims to help manage daily symptoms (e.g., dysphoric mood states), improve medication adherence and identify potential environmental stressors. Findings from prior clinical trials also link CBT to higher social functioning, reduced mood fluctuations and improved ability to cope with adverse mood experiences.

CBT lessens the total duration of affective episodes and has been linked to reductions in depressive symptoms and negative emotional states, as well as increased quality of life. Studies comparing PE to CBT have found no significant difference between the two therapies; however, given PE can be administered at a lower cost than CBT, it may be a more accessible therapy option for many, or offered first before CBT. Recent studies have supported the efficacy of combined CBT and PE programs. For example, a combined CBT-PE program was found to contribute to fewer hospitalizations, fewer anxiety symptoms and increased social-occupational functioning. However, online combined CBT-PE programs have not shown significant group differences, but this may be due to certain design characteristics, e.g., the control groups being offered similarly helpful material.[5]

Interpersonal and Social Rhythm Therapy

IPSRT is one of the first psychosocial treatments created specifically for BD and centers on the relationship between mood and circadian systems. Increasing the regularity of patients' daily routines (e.g., meal times and sleep–wake cycles) is thought to strengthen the circadian systems thereby preventing the recurrence of mood episodes and resulting in euthymia. In addition to promoting stable daily routines, it also targets areas implicated in relapse such as medication non-adherence and interpersonal stress. Group-based IPSRT has been found to reduce functional impairment, improve depressive symptomatology and enhance social rhythm stability in non-randomized clinical trials. IPSRT has been the focus of fewer controlled studies; however, recent data did find this was superior to treatment as usual in BD, with earlier studies suggesting IPSRT may be helpful for this condition.[6]

Dialectical Behavior Therapy

DBT was originally designed for borderline personality disorder as it targets emotional dysfunction, suicidality and self-harm behaviors. It has been found effective in reducing hospitalizations, enhancing treatment adherence and improving overall social functioning in adults with borderline personality disorder. Given severe mood disorders involve similar affective dysfunctions, recent clinical trials have explored the potential of DBT as an efficacious psychosocial treatment for the said conditions. In view of the data on DBT to manage suicidality and emotional dysregulation in other clinical populations, it is an excellent modality to apply to BD and MDD. Indeed, the preliminary data are quite promising. Specifically, DBT has been found to reduce both depressive and manic/hypomanic symptoms as well as to improve emotional dysregulation in individuals with BD.[7]

Mindfulness-Based Cognitive Therapy

MBCT aims to develop a nonjudgmental awareness of a patient's distressing thoughts, feelings and sensations by integrating mindfulness-based meditation practices with cognitive therapy. MBCT differs from CBT in that it encourages the individual to view negative thoughts as fleeting mental events rather than as facts. MBCT had very promising findings in reducing stress and improving quality of life in other clinical populations by increasing mind and body awareness, suggesting it could be useful for patients with severe affective disturbances. Indeed, MBCT has been found to be effective in reducing depressive symptoms and anxiety for such individuals. For instance, a non-randomized study found that bipolar patients (N = 12) who received 12 group sessions of MBCT exhibited significant pre- to post-treatment increases in mindfulness, emotional regulation, psychological well-being, positive affect and psychosocial functioning as well as significant decreases in rumination, worry, attentional difficulties and depressive symptoms.[8]

Family Therapies

These may be especially useful for individuals whose mood episodes are strongly influenced by and closely tied to their family relationships. In particular, FFT increases the number of days well, yields faster recovery from baseline depression as well as fewer weeks spent in a depressive episode and a more favorable trajectory for depressive symptoms, with reductions in family conflict. Importantly, the FFT studies have also yielded interesting findings with regards to how family factors moderate outcomes. For example, FFT is especially effective for families with dysfunctional communication styles. Families with high levels of expressed emotion (EE) would especially benefit from FFT as compared to psychoeducation, whereas families with low EE benefit equally from these treatments. Such findings highlight the importance of examining the family dynamics of an individual seeking treatment for his/her mood disorder, because patients coming from highly critical or emotionally over-involved families may especially benefit from family therapy. On the other hand, if a clinic has limited resources, individuals coming from families with low levels of expressed emotion and emotional over-involvement may not necessarily need family therapy to improve depressive symptoms. Other family therapies have been associated with lowered hospitalization rates and improvements in social functioning as well as in relatives' overall burden. As with CBT and PE, a recent study combined family therapy with several other psychotherapies (i.e., IPSRT, mindfulness, CBT, PE) with promising acceptability and efficacy findings.[9]

Future Directions in Research on Psychological Treatments

Taken together, DBT and MBCT might present some of the most interesting areas of future research for managing subthreshold symptoms and increasing the number of days well for individuals with mood disorders. However, one point to consider is how effective MBCT would be for individuals with more severe depressive symptoms, given most of the studies have only included individuals in remission or mild dysphoria. One possibility is that asking individuals to engage in skills that require intense self-reflection may encourage rumination or increased focus on negative cognitions. In contrast to rumination, MBCT asks individuals to be focused in the present moment and become aware of their thoughts and feelings in an open but nonjudgmental way. Individuals can acknowledge negative happenings but are taught to see them as passing events, which is thought to decrease rumination. Therefore, further research on MBCT in more symptomatic individuals with mood disorders is warranted.[10]

Other areas of future research include managing the leading cause of mortality in individuals with mood disorders, i.e., cardiovascular disease. For example, the Nutrition, Exercise and Wellness Treatment (NEW Tx) for overweight bipolar individuals is an 18-session, 20-week CBT-based treatment for lifestyle changes that also includes motivational interviewing techniques (sufficient sleep, reduced substance and nicotine use). Data from two pilot studies of the NEW Tx program are promising. Specifically, results from the initial pilot groups showed improvements in their quality of life, depressive symptoms and weight, with participants adding over 100 minutes of weekly exercise. A small follow-up study found weekly exercise duration more than tripled over the course of the study with subjects also experiencing improvements in depressive symptoms and life functioning. Further, patients' daily calories, sugar intake and weight decreased and serum cholesterol and triglycerides were reduced over the study duration.[11]

Another area of future research is applying the Unified Protocol for Trans-diagnostic Treatment of Emotional Disorders (UP). Rooted in PE and CBT, UP is based on the premise that individuals with anxiety and mood disorders tend to perceive emotional experiences as unpredictable and aversive and are vulnerable to more heightened affectivity than healthy controls. UP aims to identify and target the cognitive and physiological cues that contribute to maladaptive behavioral response patterns. Through extinction learning, these forms of responding are replaced with more adaptive patterns. In a replicated case series of UP for BD with comorbid anxiety, patients reported improvements in mood and affective symptomatology which provided them with a feeling of success and mastery in cognitive and behavioral decision-making.[12]

Conclusion

Several psychotherapy interventions – PE, CBT, family therapies, DBT and MBCT – are effective in improving affective symptoms and are an important component of the treatment program when administered in conjunction with pharmacotherapy. However, at this stage it is not known which treatment to try first and for whom. It is very likely that certain people (and families) will be more suited for different interventions. For example, individuals with fewer affective episodes may be well matched for CBT, whereas those higher in intrinsic motivation may be better for lifestyle interventions. In addition, a recent study using a cluster analysis of 135 symptomatic individuals with BD found that illness onset, number of previous episodes and illness duration significantly influenced response to psychotherapy. This suggests that it is important that clinicians collect comprehensive information about their patients' illness history before deciding on the most appropriate treatment modality. As a final note, mental health practitioners continue to face the dilemma of dissemination: there is higher demand for these empirically based treatments than there are skilled therapists to implement delivery. Thus, it is important to continue to explore possible solutions from creating better online interventions to increase direct access to patients, as well as to develop effective virtual training programs for therapists. In short, there are psychotherapy modalities that improve the overall outcome for mood disorders; the need is to personalize them and increase access.

Electroconvulsive Therapy

Introduction

Electroconvulsive therapy (ECT) was initiated about 80 years ago in Italy, when for the first time, Cerletti and Bini used electricity to evoke convulsive seizures in a patient experiencing a mixed state with psychotic symptoms. This patient then exhibited an improvement after a single treatment, recovered after 11 treatments, and was found to be in remission at a one-year follow-up. Since then, ECT remains the most commonly used physical treatment for mood disorders, with high effectiveness for the acute management of depressive, manic and mixed episodes. In such patients ECT is helpful in managing severe episodes, suicidality and drug resistance, and its actual availability as an efficacious treatment is very much needed. Further, the application of a modality that causes remission of depressive symptoms without destabilizing the mood is extremely desirable.[13] For these important reasons ECT remains the treatment of choice in emergency situations, and every major psychiatric unit has provisions for the administration of this treatment. Next, the use of ECT is examined in different phases of mood disorders in the light of available evidence. Figure 11.3 is a diagrammatic rendition of the utility of ECT in severe and life-threatening situations, and also illustrates its prophylactic potential in the maintenance treatment of mood disorders.

Depressive Episodes

Although there are numerous studies supporting the effectiveness of ECT for the treatment of severe and refractory depression, most of these studies involve samples of patients experiencing MDD, whereas its use in the management of BD type I and II is less extensively examined. This is particularly surprising as a large body of evidence supports the existence of major differences in the response to antidepressant drugs between unipolar and bipolar depression patients. In addition to being poorly effective, treatment of bipolar depression with antidepressants has been associated with manic switching, induction of mixed states and cycle acceleration. These phenomena are more

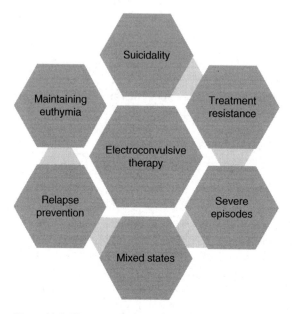

Figure 11.3 Electroconvulsive therapy as a promising strategy in mood disorders

Both major depressive disorder (MDD) and bipolar disorder (BD) can be life-threatening conditions, as increasing severity of episodes predisposes to suicidal ideation and attempts. Phenomena like rapid cycling, mixed states and psychosis greatly multiply this risk. Electroconvulsive therapy (ECT) is a fast acting and efficacious modality which is invaluable in such situations. Once euthymia is achieved, ECT can be used in a prophylactic manner to prevent future episodes and maintain remission.

commonly associated with tricyclic antidepressants than selective serotonin reuptake inhibitors (SSRIs), although the former are likely more effective for severe melancholic depression, which is commonly associated with BD.[14]

ECT seems to display similar efficacy for bipolar depression and MDD, and several studies revealed similar levels of symptomatic and functional recovery between these patients. Other studies reported MDD patients were more likely to exhibit marked improvement than BD patients. In contrast, a faster response and fewer required treatments were reported for BD patients compared with MDD patients, among those treated for severe episodes or depressive psychoses. A revealing prospective study explored the response of patients experiencing MDD or BD type I or II to ECT using a sample of patients resistant to pharmacological treatment. All groups (MDD, BD II and BD I) exhibited a significant improvement after the ECT course: the global response rate was 94.1% for MDD, 79.1% for BD II, and 67.4% for BD I. Concerning depressive symptoms, the remission rate (Hamilton Rating Scale for Depression [HRSD] ≤ 8) was 70.5% for MDD, 56.7% for BD II, and 65.3% for BD I. The MDD patients exhibited the best response and symptomatic improvement after the

ECT course. In contrast, the BD I patients were less responsive than either the MDD or BD II patients and exhibited greater residual manic and psychotic symptoms and less complete symptomatic improvement.[15]

A prospective study of a large clinical sample showed diagnosis is not a predictive factor of the response rate to an ECT course. This was greater than 60% for both unipolar and bipolar depression patients within the same time frame and with approximately the same number of treatments. The risk for switching to hypomania/mania during an ECT course was very low; thus, the authors suggested a re-evaluation of the treatment strategies for MDD and BD.[16] Finally, data regarding the relative efficacy of unilateral (UL) and bilateral (BL) ECT for the treatment of BD are scarce; however, it is likely that, as in MDD, BL electrode placement may be more effective than UL electrode placement.

In conclusion, ECT seems to display similar efficacy for both MDD and bipolar depression, with few differences in the rapidity of response and residual symptoms. The dissimilarities might be related to other course characteristics such as the duration of the episode and inter-episodic symptoms, rather than the episode itself. The literature reviewed and the meta-analysis results suggest ECT may be more effective than antidepressant drugs for the treatment of bipolar depression, particularly for medication refractory cases.[17] However, randomized comparisons between ECT and medications are lacking, and further investigation is required to clarify this issue.

Electroconvulsive Therapy for Manic/Mixed Episodes

The efficacy of ECT for mania has been widely documented for a long time, although most of these reports are of uncontrolled and retrospective studies. The few prospective studies have reported high response rates, up to 92 to 94% of cases.[18] ECT is considered as the first-line treatment option specifically for severe mania associated with life-threatening physical exhaustion, and the so-called "delirious mania". In addition, patients exhibiting mania with rapid cycling may be particularly unresponsive to medications, and ECT may represent an effective alternative treatment. In clinical practice, the treatments of choice for acute mania are mood stabilizers and antipsychotic drugs, whereas ECT is considered as the second-/third-line option for treatment-resistant patients. Other than medication resistance, few attempts have been made to examine the clinical features predictive of a response in acutely manic patients. One study suggested symptoms of anger, irritability and suspiciousness were associated with poor ECT outcome. In this respect, some overlap may exist between the clinical features predictive of the responses to ECT and lithium, as both are highly effective in classical, euphoric mania.[19] ECT has been demonstrated to display superior efficacy than sham-ECT, as well as to chlorpromazine and haloperidol. An eight-week comparative study failed to detect significant differences between lithium and ECT treatment in a sample of 34 hospitalized manic patients. In this study, however, all patients were first treated with UL ECT with the option of switching to BL ECT after at least six UL treatments without improvement. Furthermore, two double-blind randomized controlled trials (RCTs) revealed bifrontal ECT was faster than bitemporal and was associated with fewer cognitive side effects.[20]

Unlike that for bipolar depression and mania, the efficacy of ECT for mixed states (ME) is less extensively studied for several reasons. ME are often underdiagnosed because of inadequate diagnostic delimitation, and misdiagnosed because of their pleomorphic clinical presentation. Consequently, many patients experiencing ME are included in samples of schizophrenic or manic patients treated with ECT, and because of this bias, literature data are disappointingly limited. Furthermore, likely because of the limited evidence available, the use of ECT to treat ME is not specifically mentioned by several clinical practice guidelines for the treatment of mood disorders. In retrospective studies, ECT has been demonstrated to be effective for the treatment of ME, with response rates of up to 68% and a significant reduction in the severity of both depressive and manic symptoms.[21]

In a chart review, the ECT response was compared in 38 bipolar depressed, 5 manic and 10 ME patients. All groups exhibited high response rates: 76% in the depression group, 100% in the manic group and 80% in the ME group. The ME group displayed a higher number of days of hospitalization (30 versus 19) and a higher number of ECT sessions (mean, 9.3 versus 7.0) compared with the depression group. These results indirectly suggested that ME are more difficult to treat and may take longer for response to occur than "purely" depressive or manic episodes.[22] In a more recent prospective study, 96 drug-resistant BD type I patients, 46 displaying depression and 50 exhibiting ME, received ECT treatment. The patients showing ME demonstrated a good response to ECT at rates comparable to those detected for bipolar depression (66.0% versus 69.6%). However, the final Young Mania Rating Scale (YMRS), Brief Psychiatric Rating Scale (BPRS) total and psychotic cluster sub-scores were higher in the ME group than in the depression group. The only other difference was that ME subjects reported more residual agitation and functional impairment compared with the purely depressive patients.[23]

Only in one study, patients exhibiting ME displayed a greater reduction in depressive symptoms, BPRS activation factor and overall psychopathology than patients showing bipolar depression. The response rates at the endpoint were 56% for the mixed mania patients and 26% for the bipolar depression patients. In this study, the number of responses among patients exhibiting bipolar depression was particularly low, and the authors did not clearly report the ECT dosing method used. It is possible that because of an inadequate procedure, the efficacy of ECT may have been compromised.[24] In conclusion, ECT should be considered as a viable alternative treatment for patients exhibiting severe mania or ME who do not respond to conventional pharmacologic management. Compared with subjects who have purely depressive episodes, patients with ME are more difficult to treat, may develop more residual symptoms and may take longer to respond.

Maintenance Electroconvulsive Therapy

For patients exhibiting remission of an acute mood episode after an ECT course, the efficacy of continued ECT sessions has been documented since 1940. However, primarily because of the public and professional stigma regarding ECT, this treatment modality is underused and consequently poorly studied. This situation has led to the paradoxical conclusion by the National Institute for Health and Care Excellence (NICE) that they did not "recommend ECT as a maintenance therapy in depressive illness" because "the long-term benefits and risks have not been clearly established" despite a positive indication by the American Psychiatry Association. Recently, strategies to prolong remission after ECT treatment have been proposed. Symptom-Titrated, Algorithm-Based Longitudinal ECT is a novel patient-focused approach to individualize the ECT treatment schedule. Its aim is to adapt the ECT schedule to symptom fluctuations to prevent over treatment for people who do not need it and to maintain remission for people who might have otherwise relapsed using a rigid dosing schedule. The effectiveness of this approach has been demonstrated based on open prospective observations and should be examined using RCTs.[25]

In MDD, continuation ECT (c-ECT) and maintenance ECT (m-ECT) have been used to prevent relapse and recurrence of depression either alone or in conjunction with pharmacological treatment. There have been no RCTs of m-ECT specifically for BD, but some studies of c-ECT and m-ECT included BD patients. Several naturalistic observations suggested c-ECT and m-ECT may be a useful tool to stabilize chronic BD patients by reducing the admission rate or the number of days spent in the hospital. With the introduction of ultra-brief pulse width stimulation and the improvement of anesthetic procedures, the side effect profile of modern ECT has been vastly reduced, and its safety further improved. Conversely, in recent years, the wide use of polypharmacy for the long-term treatment of mood disorders has become a rule, despite the increasing evidence of serious metabolic, cardiac, neurologic and cognitive side effects. These issues are broadly relevant to the effort to introduce ECT into evidence-based management of the acute and long-term treatment of MDD and BD. RCTs comparing ECT treatment with pharmacological treatments are necessary to clarify the relative efficacy and safety of ECT for preventing recurrence and relapse associated with mood disorders.[26]

Conclusion

ECT can be considered as a mood stabilizing treatment in BD patients. In the instance of MDD, it is highly efficacious in severe, treatment refractory episodes and m-ECT is useful in relapse prevention. Unfortunately, the current guidelines and, consequently, clinical practice consider ECT to be a "last resort" treatment. As a consequence, a large proportion of patients experiencing affective disturbances are treated for a long time with different types of psychotropic medications, often in combination, before receiving ECT. This worldwide practice increases the risk of mood destabilization and chronic complications and reduces the probability of recovery for many patients who could potentially respond well if timely treated with ECT.

Chronobiological Therapy for Mood Disorders

Introduction

Despite an array of empirically validated pharmacological interventions, only 50 to 70% of patients respond to their first antidepressant treatment and less than 40% achieve remission. Most antidepressant drugs show a delayed therapeutic effect which is linked with early dropout and increased suicide risk; moreover, these agents are associated with numerous side effects and drug–drug interactions. Besides, the use of antidepressant drugs is not always advisable both in specific medical conditions and during pregnancy, in the light of safety concerns for the developing fetus and of possible anxiety-like behaviors in adulthood after prenatal antidepressant exposure.[27] Indeed, new effective and safe antidepressant therapies are still needed. Despite recent findings in pharmacology, new classes of drugs are not yet ready for clinical use in the treatment of depression.

Chronobiological therapies for mood disorders include manipulation of the sleep–wake cycle such as sleep deprivation and sleep phase advance, and the controlled exposure to light and darkness. Their antidepressant efficacy can overcome drug resistance and targets the core depressive symptoms including suicidality, thus making them significant options to be tried either alone or in conjunction with pharmacotherapy.[28] The specific pattern of mood change observed with chronobiological therapies is characterized by a rapid and sustained response, effect sizes are the same as reported for the most efficacious psychiatric treatments, but side effects are usually marginal or absent. New treatment protocols are developed to adapt them in different clinical settings. Therefore, this section deals with the general principles of clinical chronobiology and the latest findings in this rapidly developing field are highlighted. Figure 11.4 is helpful in understanding the usefulness of chronobiological therapies in the treatment of mood disorders across the entire spectrum.

Sleep Deprivation

Sleep deprivation (SD) shows a rapid antidepressant effect in every depressive syndrome, with a better efficacy having been found when treating melancholic and bipolar depression. Neither demographic nor illness characteristics appear to predict response, which tends to occur across the board. The core depressive symptoms are the first targets of SD, and the rapid improvement essentially includes suicidal thinking and planning, an effect closely similar to that of ketamine infusion and possibly due to a similar immediate dampening of glutamatergic N-methyl D-aspartate (NMDA) neurotransmission.[29] Safety concerns are

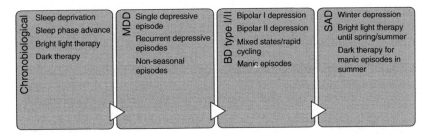

Figure 11.4 Chronobiological therapy across the spectrum of mood disorders

Chronobiological strategies, e.g., bright light therapy, were first employed for seasonal affective disorder (SAD), but now these techniques are being adapted for use in the entire spectrum of mood disorders. For instance, in major depressive disorder (MDD) various procedures are used to induce remission in non-seasonal episodes partially responsive to pharmacotherapy. Patients with bipolar disorder type I or II (BD I/II) achieve remission in depressive symptoms without switching into manic or hypomanic episodes and this is particularly valuable in cases with medication refractory depression. See text for further details.

minimal, but given that SD can trigger seizures, it should be carefully monitored in patients affected by epilepsy. Contrary to antidepressant drugs, which show long response latencies, SD shows a rapid (within 24–48 h) reversal of depressive symptoms. When treating bipolar depressed patients with repeated total SD (three cycles in a week), a 4.85% switch rate into easily controlled mania was observed. This rate is similar to that observed when using placebo and much lower than that linked with use of antidepressant drugs (15 to 25%).[30]

It is still unclear how many hours of SD are needed to achieve its full antidepressant effect. Usually, the wake period starts in the morning after regular awakening and lasts about 36 hours until the evening of the day after (total SD), but it can also start with an awakening within the second half of the night and include the following day (partial SD), with marginal reductions in efficacy in respect to total SD. This approach was reported as better tolerated in some studies, and protocols with repeated partial SD, once or twice a week, have been proposed for the continued treatment of patients, or even as a prophylactic treatment to sustain response and prevent relapses.[31] Focusing on the possibility that a short nap can block the antidepressant effects of SD, controversial results have been found. Indeed, while some studies reported a mood worsening, both after napping and even after subjectively unrecognized microsleeps, others reported napping did not change mood in responders and even ameliorated mood in nonresponders. Remarkably, responders to SD seem to adapt to sleep loss without the need of the huge homeostatic sleep rebound which is observed in nonresponders, and which precedes the early relapse.[32]

The clinical usefulness of SD in the treatment of mood disorders has been questioned by the short duration of its antidepressant effects, with up to 80% of SD responders relapsing (though mostly not completely) after the recovery sleep night. In the following days, a trend of progressive worsening is shown by patients who often reach a clinical severity similar to that seen at baseline. If other combined treatments are not added to SD, only the 5% of early respond-ers will maintain a stable euthymia after restoration of normal sleep. To pre-vent relapse, repetition of SD alone was proven useless, because after eventual discontinuation patients relapsed in the same proportion and a tolerance to the therapeutic effects was reported. The concomitant use of other chrono-therapeutic interventions such as light therapy (LT) or sleep phase advance (SPA) has been proven to be effective at preventing the early relapse after SD. Bright LT was used during and after SD and it was found not only to maintain the clinical improvement generated by both partial and repeated total SD but also to increase the antidepressant effect.[33] The efficacy of SPA in pre-venting SD early relapses was proven using two different schedules: one week and three days. A one-week schedule was employed during early studies: one night of total sleep deprivation (TSD) was administered to patients; the day after, the first recovery night, bedtime started at 5 p.m. and was delayed daily by 1 h until reaching a bedtime of 11 p.m. The three-day schedule, which was proven to be effective in preventing relapses comparable to the one-week schedule, had been proposed during more recent studies. After one night of TSD, bedtime started as well at 5 p.m. during the first recovery night, but then it was delayed daily by 2 h until the conventional bedtime. In recent years, a triple chronotherapy protocol (combined TSD, SPA, and bright LT) was introduced. A single TSD night followed by a three-day scheduled SPA and three or five days of bright LT was found to have sustained antidepressant effects.[34] Remarkably, these protocols showed similar efficacy and effect sizes irrespective of ethnic differences and associated treatments, with a synergis-tic effect for standard antidepressants. Lithium salts were found not only to enhance the acute antidepressant efficacy of SD in bipolar depression, but also to prevent both acute and delayed relapses. The use of combined repeated SD and LT together with a concomitant administration of lithium salts could then maintain clinical remission, with the most severe symptoms disappearing rapidly and euthymic states maintained for months.[35]

Sleep Phase Advance Therapy

SPA therapy consists of advancing the timing of the sleep–wake cycle. Antidepressant effects of this intervention have been suggested by the theory linking depression to a misalignment in the sleep–wake cycle, the circadian clock and biological rhythms. While SPA was shown to ameliorate depres-sion, in non-depressed subjects, mood was found to worsen after an acute phase delay in sleep. This mood worsening even generated a depressive syn-drome in a minority of predisposed subjects. These findings are in agreement with demonstrated relationships between rhythm phase shifts generated by transcontinental flights and mood episodes. Indeed, when passengers flew from east to west (having a consequent phase delay in circadian rhythms), they were shown to have an increased risk of depression incidence while the opposite was true for hypomania. SPA was found to improve the antidepressant effects of drug treatments and it was extensively used to improve and sustain response after SD. While SPA therapy administered for 2–3 weeks has been found to produce a clinical improvement in about 75% of treated patients, SPA alone has never caught on in clinical settings, probably because a phase advanced sleep schedule does not match with social and environmental cues and expectations.[36]

Light Therapy

The therapeutic use of LT started in the 1980s and for decades it remained mainly confined to the treatment of seasonal affective disorder (SAD), despite early studies specifically addressing the treatment of non-seasonal depression. LT is now acknowledged a powerful antidepressant which can be used with the same efficacy and indications as antidepressant drugs. LT for SAD was developed to extend daytime photoperiod and counteract winter darkness. SAD is a form of depression that has a seasonal pattern, which typically occurs in the autumn and winter with remission in the spring or summer. The prevalence of SAD is 2–5% in the general population in temperate climates. In addition to general symptoms of depression such as depressed mood and diminished interest or pleasure, patients with SAD often show atypical vegetative symptoms including hyperphagia (particularly carbohydrate rich foods), weight gain and hypersomnia. Since the lack of sunlight during the winter is related to SAD, LT is used to mimic a summer photoperiod. LT is now considered to be the first-line treatment for SAD because of its low side effect profile and high response rate. A well-cited narrative review showed remission rates of up to 67% in patients with mild SAD and 40% in severe SAD.[37]

The conventional LT system consists of a set of white fluorescent bulbs installed in a box with a diffusing screen that filters out UV light. During LT sessions, patients sit in front of a light box mounted on a table with their eyes open. The recommended initial dose is 10,000 lux for 30 min/day in the early morning. Lower intensities can also be effective, but they need substantially longer exposure durations, e.g., 2500 lux for 2 h/day. The effects of LT do not persist after discontinuation; therefore, treatment is continued until the time of usual spontaneous remission in the spring or summer. LT is generally well tolerated and well accepted by patients. Adverse effects may include headache, eyestrain, nausea and agitation, but these are usually transient and mild.

LT is an efficacious treatment not only for SAD but also for non-seasonal major depression with effect sizes equivalent to those in most antidepressant pharmacotherapy trials. Double-blind, placebo-controlled studies found LT combined with an SSRI lead to more rapid (within a week) and more profound (by approximately 30%) improvement in patients with non-seasonal depression than drugs alone.[38] The finding of these studies was consistent with the earliest reports and suggested the usefulness of LT as an adjunct therapy in treating non-seasonal depression, especially in the initial treatment phase. In the course of ultra-rapid cycling BD, LT given at midday and not in the morning, could also be tailored to counteract depressive swings without exacerbating mania. Benefits can be obtained in the most severe, chronic and refractory cases of depression in both MDD and BD. A report on four treated cases raised concerns about the possibility of triggering manic switches in BD, but studies on hundreds of treated bipolar depressed patients over 30 years ruled it out and confirmed efficacy.[39]

The therapeutic response to LT critically depends on time of delivery relative to personal circadian phase, which is determined by the onset of melatonin secretion. A study found bright light administered 7.5–9.5 h after evening melatonin onset produced twice the remission rate (80 versus 40%) of light presented 9.5–11 h after melatonin onset and proposed to administer bright light about 8.5 h after melatonin onset for obtaining maximum therapeutic effect. However, it is not always practicable to directly measure melatonin onset in daily clinical practice. A practical solution is found in the Morningness–Eveningness Questionnaire score, which strongly correlates with melatonin onset. Using this questionnaire, optimal administration time of LT can be determined without direct measurement of melatonin.[40]

Although the exact mechanism of action of LT in treating SAD has remained unclear, it is assumed LT exerts its therapeutic effect by restoring circadian rhythm to a normal phase position. The circadian rhythm of core body temperature, cortisol and melatonin secretion is known to be phase-delayed in most SAD patients. Bright light in the morning, which causes phase advance of endogenous circadian rhythms, could correct misalignment between endogenous rhythms and sleep–wake cycle, resulting in clinical improvement. The treatment response usually begins two to four days after the start of LT, and it is completed within two weeks. If there is still no response, evening light (7–9 p.m.), which causes a phase delay of endogenous rhythms, should be tried since a small subgroup of SAD patients may be phase-advanced.[41]

Dark Therapy

A single pilot trial showed that while exposure to light is antidepressant, exposure to dark can reduce manic symptoms as rapidly as antipsychotic drugs, when administered during the first weeks of the manic episode and patients might be more sensitive to chronobiological interventions.[42] Also, the continuous mood swings of rapid cyclers appear to stabilize when maintaining a regular light–dark rhythm with an increased darkness period. This promising approach, which could reduce the need for antipsychotic drugs and lead to shorter hospitalizations, is still awaiting evaluation in randomized trials. Future research will clarify if the dark therapy approach might be clinically useful alone or combined with LT and SD to improve clinical efficacy.

Conclusion

Chronobiological therapies in treating mood disorders are characterized by rapid and sustained effects, when combining the modalities among themselves or with drugs. Effect sizes are the same as reported for the most efficacious psychiatric treatments, but the latency of action is smaller and side effects are usually marginal or absent. Chronobiological therapies are a viable treatment option in patients for whom drug therapy may be contraindicated, such as pregnant women, elderly people and patients with severe medical diseases. In conclusion, chronobiological therapies could fill the gap left by traditional antidepressant drugs in the treatment of mood disorders, and the manipulation of biological and circadian rhythms should serve as the starting point for developing more efficacious therapeutic interventions.

Summary Points

- Modern psychopharmacological agents have better tolerability and acceptability than earlier medications.
- Nonetheless, there are several caveats associated with their use, for example metabolic side effects, sexual dysfunction, cognitive problems, and relative contraindications during pregnancy and lactation.
- These limitations result in poor compliance from patients and less than optimal control of psychiatric syndromes.
- As such non-pharmacological interventions have attracted a great deal of interest as they do not carry the abovementioned stipulations and can be safely given even in medically unwell populations.
- In mood disorder patients, manual-based psychotherapies are delivered in a structured manner and are particularly helpful in relapse prevention in conjunction with pharmacotherapy.
- ECT is a brain stimulation technique, introduced almost 80 years ago and widely used in all major psychiatric facilities.
- ECT is regarded as an essential tool in treating severe, treatment-refractory affective episodes and in suicidal patients, when an urgent response is required.
- Continuation and maintenance ECT is presently being pursued with renewed interest in preventing affective recurrences in major mood disorders and sustaining euthymia.
- A review of the extant literature shows that in severe mood disturbances ECT is the treatment of choice when compared to other brain stimulation techniques.
- Chronobiological therapies, which include SD, SPA and LT, work by modulating the daily circadian rhythms and are being followed by new impetus in the treatment of major mood disorders.
- Future developments in these areas can greatly benefit patients who have refractory mood disorders, or in whom psychotherapeutic drugs are relatively contraindicated.

References

1) Aaltonen K, Näätänen P, Heikkinen M, Koivisto M, Baryshnikov I, Karpov B, et al. Differences and similarities of risk factors for suicidal ideation and attempts among patients with depressive or bipolar disorders. J Affect Disord 2016;193:318–330.

2) Sim K, Lau WK, Sim J, Sum MY, Baldessarini RJ. Prevention of relapse and recurrence in adults with major depressive disorder: systematic review and meta-analyses of controlled trials. Int J Neuropsychopharmacol 2015;19:pyv076.

3) Guidi J, Tomba E, Fava GA. The sequential integration of pharmacotherapy and psychotherapy in the treatment of major depressive disorder: a meta-analysis of the sequential model and a critical review of the literature. Am J Psychiatry 2016;173:128–137.

4) Buntrock C, Ebert DD, Lehr D, Smit F, Riper H, Berking M, et al. Effect of a web-based guided self-help intervention for prevention of major depression in adults with subthreshold depression: a randomized clinical trial. JAMA 2016;315:1854–1863.

5) Arnberg FK, Linton SJ, Hultcrantz M, Heintz E, Jonsson U. Internet-delivered psychological treatments for mood and anxiety disorders: a systematic review of their efficacy, safety, and cost-effectiveness. PLoS One 2014;9:e98118.

6) Haynes PL, Gengler D, Kelly M. Social rhythm therapies for mood disorders: an update. Curr Psychiatry Rep 2016;18:75.

7) Goldstein TR, Fersch-Podrat RK, Rivera M, Axelson DA, Merranko J, Yu H, et al. Dialectical behavior therapy for adolescents with bipolar disorder: results from a pilot randomized trial. J Child Adolesc Psychopharmacol 2015;25:140–149.

8) Deckersbach T, Hölzel BK, Eisner LR, Stange JP, Peckham AD, Dougherty DD, et al. Mindfulness-based cognitive therapy for nonremitted patients with bipolar disorder. CNS Neurosci Ther 2012;18:133–141.

9) West AE, Weinstein SM, Peters AT, Katz AC, Henry DB, Cruz RA, et al. Child- and family-focused cognitive-behavioral therapy for pediatric bipolar disorder: a randomized clinical trial. J Am Acad Child Adolesc Psychiatry 2014;53:1168–1178.

10) de Jong M, Peeters F, Gard T, Ashih H, Doorley J, Walker R, et al. A randomized controlled pilot study on mindfulness-based cognitive therapy for unipolar depression in patients with chronic pain. J Clin Psychiatry. 2017;[Epub ahead of print].

11) Sylvia LG, Salcedo S, Bernstein EE, Baek JH, Nierenberg AA, Deckersbach T. Nutrition, exercise, and wellness treatment in bipolar disorder: proof of concept for a consolidated intervention. Int J Bipolar Disord 2013;1:24.

12) Ellard KK, Deckersbach T, Sylvia LG, Nierenberg AA, Barlow DH. Transdiagnostic treatment of bipolar disorder and comorbid anxiety with the unified protocol: a clinical replication series. Behav Modif 2012;36:482–508.

13) Perugi G, Medda P, Toni C, Mariani MG, Socci C, Mauri M. The role of electroconvulsive therapy (ECT) in bipolar disorder: effectiveness in 522 patients with bipolar depression, mixed-state, mania and catatonic features. Curr Neuropharmacol 2017;15:359–371.

14) Liu B, Zhang Y, Fang H, Liu J, Liu T, Li L. Efficacy and safety of long-term antidepressant treatment for bipolar disorders – a meta-analysis of randomized controlled trials. J Affect Disord 2017;223:41–48.

15) Medda P, Perugi G, Zanello S, Ciuffa M, Cassano GB. Response to ECT in bipolar I, bipolar II and unipolar depression. J Affect Disord 2009;118:55–59.

16) Bailine S, Fink M, Knapp R, Petrides G, Husain MM, Rasmussen K, et al. Electroconvulsive therapy is equally effective in unipolar and bipolar depression. Acta Psychiatr Scand 2010;121:431–436.

17) Haq AU, Sitzmann AF, Goldman ML, Maixner DF, Mickey BJ. Response of depression to electroconvulsive therapy: a meta-analysis of clinical predictors. J Clin Psychiatry 2015;76:1374–1384.

18) Mohan TS, Tharyan P, Alexander J, Raveendran NS. Effects of stimulus intensity on the efficacy and safety of twice-weekly, bilateral electroconvulsive therapy (ECT) combined with antipsychotics in acute mania: a randomised controlled trial. Bipolar Disord 2009;11:126–134.

19) Bergink V, Rasgon N, Wisner KL. Postpartum psychosis: madness, mania, and melancholia in motherhood. Am J Psychiatry 2016;173:1179–1188.

20) Barekatain M, Jahangard L, Haghighi M, Ranjkesh F. Bifrontal versus bitemporal electroconvulsive therapy in severe manic patients. J ECT 2008;24:199–202.

21) Palma M, Ferreira B, Borja-Santos N, Trancas B, Monteiro C, Cardoso G. Efficacy of electroconvulsive therapy in bipolar disorder with mixed features. Depress Res Treat 2016;2016:8306071.

22) Devanand DP, Polanco P, Cruz R, Shah S, Paykina N, Singh K, et al. The efficacy of ECT in mixed affective states. J ECT 2000;16:32–37.

23) Medda P, Perugi G, Zanello S, Ciuffa M, Cassano GB. Response to ECT in bipolar I, bipolar II and unipolar depression. J Affect Disord 2009;118:55–59.

24) Ciapparelli A, Dell'Osso L, Tundo A, Pini S, Chiavacci MC, Di Sacco I, et al. Electroconvulsive therapy in medication-nonresponsive patients with mixed mania and bipolar depression. J Clin Psychiatry 2001;62:552–555.

25) Youssef NA, McCall WV. Relapse prevention after index electroconvulsive therapy in treatment-resistant depression. Ann Clin Psychiatry 2014;26:288–296.

26) Weiner RD, Reti IM. Key updates in the clinical application of electroconvulsive therapy. Int Rev Psychiatry 2017;29:54–62.

27) Hermansen TK, Melinder A. Prenatal SSRI exposure: effects on later child development. Child Neuropsychol 2015;21:543–569.

28) Dallaspezia S, Suzuki M, Benedetti F. Chronobiological therapy for mood disorders. Curr Psychiatry Rep 2015;17:95.

29) Wolf E, Kuhn M, Normann C, Mainberger F, Maier JG, Maywald S, et al. Synaptic plasticity model of therapeutic sleep deprivation in major depression. Sleep Med Rev 2016;30:53–62.

30) Salvadore G, Quiroz JA, Machado-Vieira R, Henter ID, Manji HK, Zarate CA Jr. The neurobiology of the switch process in bipolar disorder: a review. J Clin Psychiatry 2010;71:1488–1501.

31) Benedetti F, Colombo C. Sleep deprivation in mood disorders. Neuropsychobiology 2011;64:141–151.

32) Gershon A, Do D, Satyanarayana S, Shah S, Yuen LD, Hooshmand F, et al. Abnormal sleep duration associated with hastened depressive recurrence in bipolar disorder. J Affect Disord 2017;218:374–379.

33) Khalifeh AH. The effect of chronotherapy on depressive symptoms. Evidence-based practice. Saudi Med J 2017;38:457–464.

34) Echizenya M, Suda H, Takeshima M, Inomata Y, Shimizu T. Total sleep deprivation followed by sleep phase advance and bright light therapy in drug-resistant mood disorders. J Affect Disord 2013;144:28–33.

35) Benedetti F, Riccaboni R, Locatelli C, Poletti S, Dallaspezia S, Colombo C. Rapid treatment response of suicidal symptoms to lithium, sleep deprivation, and light therapy (chronotherapeutics) in drug-resistant bipolar depression. J Clin Psychiatry 2014;75:133–140.

36) Dopierała E, Rybakowski J. Sleep deprivation as a method of chronotherapy in the treatment of depression. Psychiatr Pol 2015;49:423–433.

37) Pail G, Huf W, Pjrek E, Winkler D, Willeit M, Praschak-Rieder N, et al. Bright-light therapy in the treatment of mood disorders. Neuropsychobiology 2011;64:152–162.

38) Lam RW, Levitt AJ, Levitan RD, Michalak EE, Cheung AH, Morehouse R, et al. Efficacy of bright light treatment, fluoxetine, and the combination in patients with nonseasonal major depressive disorder: a randomized clinical trial. JAMA Psychiatry 2016;73:56–63.

39) Penders TM, Stanciu CN, Schoemann AM, Ninan PT, Bloch R, Saeed SA. Bright light therapy as augmentation of pharmacotherapy for treatment of depression: a systematic review and meta-analysis. Prim Care Companion CNS Disord 2016;18.

40) Knapen SE, Gordijn MC, Meesters Y. The relation between chronotype and treatment outcome with light therapy on a fixed time schedule. J Affect Disord 2016;202:87–90.

41) Bais B, Kamperman AM, van der Zwaag MD, Dieleman GC, Harmsen van der Vliet-Torij HW, Bijma HH, et al. Bright light therapy in pregnant women with major depressive disorder: study protocol for a randomized, double-blind, con-trolled clinical trial. BMC Psychiatry 2016;16:381.

42) Crowe M, Porter R. Inpatient treatment for mania: a review and rationale for adjunctive interventions. Aust N Z J Psychiatry 2014;48:716–721.

Index

Note: Page numbers in *italics* and **bold** denote figures and tables, respectively.